More Praise for *100 Questions and Answers Wellness and Vitality: A Practical Guide for Sexual Fulfillment*

This is a timely, important, comprehensive, educ... Dr. Krychman provides important information ... encouraging the reader to identify and dispel m... to diversity. It is sufficiently sophisticated to als... in the area. Dr. Krychman takes the reader on a t... cultural factors known to influence women's sex... resources, helpful tips, and encouragement, an... ranging from basic science to new age comple... woman with distressing sexual dysfunction and ... who wishes to further improve her state of sexual health. Readers, regardless of age, menopausal status, health, relationship status, and even gender, will benefit from this excellent collection of answers to 100 common sexual questions.

—**Lori A. Brotto, PhD, R Psych**
Assistant Professor
University of British Columbia
Department of Obstetrics & Gynaecology

Among the extensive selection of books about female sexual health available today, this is by far the most humanly written, understandable, and comprehensive. Dr Krychman enlightens his readers by discussing current sexuality research and delights his readers with his honest, sensitive and practical approach to making sexual relationships work. My patients will love this book—I can't recommend it too highly!

—**Dr. Susan Kellogg-Spadt**
Medical Sexologist
Co-Director: The Pelvic & Sexual Health Institute of Philadelphia

This is the book for every woman who cares about her sexual health and wellness. It covers answers to questions women are looking for. A must-have resource.

—**Lisa Martinez, RN, JD**
Executive Director and Founder
The Women's Sexual Health Foundation

Dr. Krychman really does answer all those sex questions that you were afraid to ask. With a combination of good humour and sound scientific knowledge, he discusses the physical, the psychological, the spiritual and the downright strange. This book is both eminently readable and intriguing, and also offers sound, practical advice. It covers controversial issues in an accessible and non-judgemental way, and debunks many myths. Finally, it is not just for women; their physicians and most men might learn many useful things from it—I certainly have.

—**Dr. John Dean, Sexual Physician**
St Peter's Sexual Medicine Centre, London
President, International Society for Sexual Medicine

This complete resource on women's sexuality provides understandable explanations, practical advice, and creative solutions to the complex, multidimensional problem of female sexual dysfunction, with the goal of maintaining lifelong intimacy and sexual pleasure. Valuable reading for all women regardless of age, background, or current situation.

–Anita H. Clayton, MD
Professor of Psychiatry & Neurobehavioral Sciences and
Clinical Obstetrics & Gynecology,
University of Virginia,
Charlottesville, VA

Michael Krychman is a medical doctor who recognizes that sex is a vital component of overall health and well-being. *Sexual Wellness*, is a comprehensive guide to women's sexual health, and it belongs on the bookshelf or nightstand of every woman (and her partner) who takes her health and sex life seriously. The question and answer format is direct and easy to read and covers topics ranging from love and sexuality, sex throughout the life cycle, and sex and chronic illness. This book is a valuable resource for laypeople and health professionals alike and is sure to pave the way for women and their doctors to routinely address sexual issues as part of their overall health care.

–Talli Y. Rosenbaum
Urogynecological Physiotherapist
AASECT Certified Sexual Counselor
Bar Ilan University Sex Therapy Program,
Tel Aviv, Israel

Women with breast cancer are generally well-treated these days but when it comes to picking up the pieces afterwards, it's often another matter.
Sexual problems are more common than we think, with treatments that often involve removal of the breast, suppression or removal of the ovaries, or anti-estrogen treatments.
Michael Krychman is right—when he says "do not be afraid of the Pandora's box . . . ignoring a problem will not make it disappear."
Michael's 100 questions and answers are right on the mark and address not only the common but also the less common and difficult issues of sexual wellness.
This is a great resource for doctors and their patients. The "pearls" he offers for treating sexual problems are a must-read!

–Prof. John Boyages, MD
Director, Breast Cancer Institute NSW, Australia

Dr. Krychman's newest book, *100 Questions and Answers About Women's Sexual Wellness and Vitality* addresses every question that any woman might pose about sex (and one or two she hasn't thought of)! It is informal in tone, encyclopedic in scope, and can be a one-stop reference guide for all women.

–Sandra Leiblum, PhD
Director, New Jersey Center for Sexual Wellness
Author of *Getting The Sex You Want:*
A Woman's Guide to Becoming Proud, Passionate and Pleased in Bed

Dr. Krychman takes the responsible physician's approach in writing this book to help women address their sexual issues. Using an easy-to-read format, he clearly, thoroughly, and understandably answers 100 of the key questions women are likely to ask. Dr. Krychman taps his wealth of sexual-medicine knowledge to give readers the equal of a private session with him. At a time when female sexual dysfunction is still dismissed by many physicians as "being in your head" Dr. Krychman is at the forefront showing that he knows these problems are real, and providing this book to help.

–Ralph Alterowitz
Founder & Co-Director
Center for Intimacy After Cancer Therapy (CIACT)
Author, *Intimacy with Impotence*

Michael L. Krychman, MD, like the center he directs, enhances the lives of patients and their partners through assessment and treatment of the physical, psychological, medical and surgical causes of sexual and intimacy concerns. For all women with questions about sex, Krychman provides clear, understandable, and meaningful answers. For women diagnosed with cancer, Kryman has always had a special message of hope and help for their survivorship.

–Michael A. Perelman, PhD
President, Society for Sex Therapy and Research
& Co-Director, Human Sexuality Program
Clinical Associate Professor of Psychiatry,
Reproductive Medicine and Urology
The NY Weill Cornell Medical Center
New York, NY

100 Questions and Answers About Women's Sexual Wellness and Vitality:
A Practical Guide for the Woman Seeking Sexual Fulfillment

Michael L. Krychman, MD, FACOG
Medical Director of Sexual Medicine, Hoag Hospital
Executive Director of the Southern California Center for Sexual Health and
Survivorship Medicine
Associate Clinical Professor University of Southern California
Associate Clinical Professor University of California, Irvine
ASSECT Certified Sexual Counselor
Sexual Addiction Specialist

JONES AND BARTLETT PUBLISHERS
Sudbury, Massachusetts
BOSTON   TORONTO   LONDON   SINGAPORE

World Headquarters

Jones and Bartlett Publishers	Jones and Bartlett Publishers	Jones and Bartlett Publishers
40 Tall Pine Drive	Canada	International
Sudbury, MA 01776	6339 Ormindale Way	Barb House, Barb Mews
978-443-5000	Mississauga, Ontario L5V 1J2	London W6 7PA
info@jbpub.com	Canada	United Kingdom
www.jbpub.com		

Jones and Bartlett's books and products are available through most bookstores and online booksellers. To contact Jones and Bartlett Publishers directly, call 800-832-0034, fax 978-443-8000, or visit our website, www.jbpub.com.

Substantial discounts on bulk quantities of Jones and Bartlett's publications are available to corporations, professional associations, and other qualified organizations. For details and specific discount information, contact the special sales department at Jones and Bartlett via the above contact information or send an email to specialsales@jbpub.com.

The authors, editor, and publisher have made every effort to provide accurate information. However, they are not responsible for errors, omissions, or for any outcomes related to the use of the contents of this book and take no responsibility for the use of the products and procedures described. Treatments and side effects described in this book may not be applicable to all people; likewise, some people may require a dose or experience a side effect that is not described herein. Drugs and medical devices are discussed that may have limited availability controlled by the Food and Drug Administration (FDA) for use only in a research study or clinical trial. Research, clinical practice, and government regulations often change the accepted standard in this field. When consideration is being given to use of any drug in the clinical setting, the healthcare provider or reader is responsible for determining FDA status of the drug, reading the package insert, and reviewing prescribing information for the most up-to-date recommendations on dose, precautions, and contraindications, and determining the appropriate usage for the product. This is especially important in the case of drugs that are new or seldom used.

Production Credits

Executive Publisher: Christopher Davis
Production Editor: Rachel Rossi
Sr. Editorial Assistant: Jessica Acox
Marketing Manager: Ilana Goddess

V. P., Manufacturing and Inventory Control: Therese Connell
Composition: Appingo Publishing Services
Printing and Binding: Malloy, Inc.
Cover Printing: Malloy, Inc.

Cover Credits
Cover Design: Kristin E. Parker
Cover Images: Elderly Couple: © Kurhan ShutterStock, Inc.
Blond Woman: © Darren Baker/ShutterStock, Inc.
Young Couple: © Dewayne Flowers/ShutterStock, Inc.
African-American Female: © iofoto/ShutterStock, Inc.

Library of Congress Cataloging-in-Publication Data
Krychman, Michael L.
  100 questions and answers about women's sexual wellness and vitality : a practical guide for the woman seeking sexual fulfillment / Michael L Krychman.
    p. cm.
  Includes bibliographical references and index.
  ISBN-13: 978-0-7637-5448-8 (alk. paper)
  ISBN-10: 0-7637-5448-X (alk. paper)
  1. Women—Health and hygiene. 2. Women—Sexual behavior. 3. Hygiene, Sexual.
  4. Gynecology—Popular works. 5. Sex instruction for women. I. Title. II. Title: One hundred questions and answers about female sexual wellness and vitality.
  RG121.K8943 2010
  613'.04244—dc22
                              2009001088
6048
Printed in the United States of America
13 12 11 10 09   10 9 8 7 6 5 4 3 2 1

For the love of my life, and the beautiful and wondrous twins Julianna and Russell: You have taught me what love and life is truly about.
Thank you for the lifelong lesson.

CONTENTS

PART ONE

Sensuality, Sexuality, Dysfunction, and Assessment

What is sexual medicine?

What is the incidence of sexual problems and why study them?

What are common sexual complaints?

More . . .

1. What is sexual medicine?

Sexual medicine means different things to different people. To some it conjures up images of intense therapy sessions delving into your sexual past and upbringing, whereas to other individuals it represents a complete medicalized approach to **sexuality**. Others still take the approach of a comprehensive yet dynamic definition. The most common definition of sexual medicine describes it as the medical discipline that embraces the study, diagnosis, and treatment of sexual health concerns of both men and women. Another interesting and thought-provoking definition is used at this author's center, the Southern California Center for Sexual Health and Survivorship Medicine located in Newport Beach. There, sexual medicine and health is described as the discipline that seeks to enhance the lives of patients and their partners through assessment and treatment of the physical, psychological, medical, and surgical causes of sexual and intimacy concerns.

Although sexual medicine is not an accepted discipline of formalized medical school study, many healthcare institutions and educational programs are embracing the notion of sexual health and intimacy as an important facet for overall patient quality of life. Sexual health involves many disciplines including urology, gynecology, psychiatry, and other fields of medical study. Many recognize that the interface of medical experience, or the mere fact of going to see a doctor, no matter what the diagnosis, often changes their relationships. Health-care teams now understand that to better serve their patients, the concept of sexual intimacy must be addressed in study and treatment.

Sexual complaints are common in both men and women, and failure to have these problems diagnosed and treated effectively can lead to both personal distress and relational disruption. Sexual complaints are independent of race, color, and creed or ethnicity. Women of all races and backgrounds are at risk for and complain of sexual issues. Although much of

Sexuality

The feelings, behaviors, and identities associated with sex.

Sexual medicine and health is described as the discipline that seeks to enhance the lives of patients and their partners through assessment and treatment of the physical, psychological, medical, and surgical causes of sexual and intimacy concerns.

ACKNOWLEDGMENTS

To Tenille, I thank you for your commitment to our healthcare team. I must thank my parents in advance for their courage and support to endure the undoubted snickers that they may encounter because their son is a sexual medicine specialist and has written a book about human sexuality. I can only hope that this book will not embarrass them too much and that they continue to be proud. For Steven, Nancy, Hailey, and Gregory, my favorite and special Aunt Ann, the Franconi family, and the others who have touched my life and have given me unconditional support, your thoughts do not go unappreciated. Dr. Susan Kellogg—I am fortunate to have you as a colleague and a special friend.

Julianna and Russell, you never cease to amaze and thrill me, I hope that one day, both of you may benefit from the information in this book and find it useful during your own personal relationships. (P.S. Just please, don't tell me about it.) To my family, who have endured the late nights and key pad banging, thanks for free passes to have time to commit to my career and writing; your support is always appreciated and does not go unnoticed.

This is not merely another book about sex or sexual function; I would hope people who read this understand there is much more to sex and relationships than the physical aspects. I hope that intimacy and connectedness resound in the pages of this book and that many will benefit in their journeys of couplehood.

No relationship is ideal or perfect. Sometimes even the clearest of relationships can become clouded, and often you can lose your way or become confused. There is not one formula for success and neither does sexual health and wellness follow a single, cookie-cutter treatment. No two couples are the same in their needs and wants. Luckily, I have been fortunate to have learned much from many of the loving and supportive couples I have come across in my years. Each has taught me something unique and special, and

I can hope to write their lessons and words of wisdom on paper. A special thank you for Paul and Muriel, Steven and Nancy, Joe and Rose, Susan and Kirk, Tom and Judy, Vera and Morty, Cammy and Olga.

I would also like to extend a thank you to all the women who are brave enough to seek out care from a sexual healthcare professional—they have the courage to demand improved quality of life and want connectedness with their loved one.

Every day during my California commute, I travel along the Pacific Coast Highway and enjoy the ocean's beauty and breezes on my way to the office. Since living in California, I have learned that the ocean can often serve as a metaphor for intimate relationships. Close connections with other people are sometimes like the ocean: sometimes they are smooth, serene, and pleasing while at other times they can be stormy, troublesome, or even frightening. But personal and life experiences have taught me that the keys to relationship success include communication, compromise, cooperation, patience, selflessness, compassion, and understanding.

I hope that this book will serve as a helpful blueprint for all women, of all ages, races, cultures, orientations, and background, so that they have the knowledge, insight, tools, and self-awareness to weather any storm.

the sexual medicine research and information readily available typically focus on the upper-middle-class Caucasian female, new data support that minority women and those of different socioeconomic classes should also be asked about, assessed, and treated for sexual complaints. Sexual health and wellness is often influenced by a variety of cultural issues. With respect to African American and other minorities and sexual wellness, there may be some barriers; disparities based on gender, race, and other factors inhibit many minority women from acquiring the tools for sexual health. These women often lack access to good medical health care let alone sexual medicine services. Sometimes negative sexual stereotypes affect sexual self-esteem and also inhibit the path to sexual awareness and wellness. For example, historical myths surviving since the time of slavery and other points in black history perpetuate falsehoods about African American women, such as the notion of their hypersexuality as well as prevailing thoughts that many women enjoy sexual activity or are "loose" or "disinhibited"; these are falsehoods that many women struggle to overcome even today.

According to the World Health Organization Report on Education and Treatment in Human Sexuality, sexual health is the integration of the somatic, emotional, intellectual, and social aspects of sexual being in ways that are positively enriching and that enhance personality, communication, and love. Sexual health should not be a privilege of the few and well insured—all women deserve access to well-qualified sexual health specialists.

Raye comments:

Sexual medicine is the specialty that deals with sexual health. It can be anything from sexual disorders to concerns with your body. Pain or low sexual interest are common problems too. I really didn't even know that it existed until a friend told me about it. I was suffering in silence and thought that I was alone. It's not true. You do not have to suffer alone; there is help available.

Sensuality, Sexuality, Dysfunction, and Assessment

2. What is the incidence of sexual problems and why study them?

It is estimated that 43% of all women suffer from some form of sexual problem or complaint.

Hypertension

High blood pressure. An abnormality in arterial blood pressure that typically results from a thickening of the blood vessel wall. It is a risk factor for many illnesses including heart attacks, heart failure, and stroke or end-stage kidney disease.

It is estimated that 43% of all women suffer from some form of sexual problem or complaint. Low desire or hypoactive sexual desire disorders are the most common forms of sexual complaint. The National Cancer Institute estimates that 40–100% of female cancer survivors suffer from sexual problems that cause personal distress. Women with any chronic medical illness including **hypertension**, diabetes, or endocrinopathies all suffer from sexual complaints. The data do support the fact that as women age, the incidence of sexual complaints increases (however, older women are less bothered by the problems than their younger counterparts are). Although many women have sexual issues and problems, many do not complain and many suffer in silence. Clearly, only women who are bothered or distressed by their sexual healthcare concerns should seek professional medical care and treatment.

According to a recent article titled "Survey Says Patients Expect Little Physician Help On Sex." published in the *Journal of the American Medical Association*:

- 85% of adults would like to discuss sexual functioning with their physician; however, they do not for many reasons.
- 71% believe their physician would not want or have the time to deal with sexual problems.
- 68% of adults are concerned about embarrassing their physician.
- 76% thought no treatment was available for their problems.

There is a need for accurate medical information concerning the diagnosis, assessment, and effective treatment of sexual complaints. Busy healthcare providers, internists, and primary care physicians can use this book as part of a comprehensive educational tool to help their patients achieve sexual satisfaction.

Interestingly, one act of **sexual intercourse** burns 200 calories or is about the equivalent of 30 minutes of jogging. Sexual intercourse is an excellent aerobic activity that improves cardiovascular health and releases endogenous endorphins (brain feel-good hormones). Sexual hormones may also influence and lead to lower rates of **depression**, anxiety, suicide, and infections and may boost immunity, which can increase longevity. Oxytocin and DHEA (which stands for dehydroepiandrosterone), two hormones that are both released during **orgasm**, may prevent breast cancer cells from developing into tumors. The Viagra-ization of America—with millions of prescriptions and users—has lead to changing cultural stereotypes of middle-aged men and women. Middle-aged women are now viewed as strong, vibrant, sexual human beings. Coupled with this cultural change in perspective on sexuality is more focus on research and emerging treatments of sexual dysfunction.

3. What are the stages of the sexual response cycle?

To discuss sexual dysfunction, a primer on human sexuality is essential. Human sexuality is not a static concept, but one that is dynamic and multidimensional. It is a product of interpersonal, biological, psychological, and cultural mechanisms that help formulate an individual's personal view of sexuality. Each individual has a personal and unique sexual schema; it is not possible to impose a singular approach and view on sexuality that applies uniformly across races, sexes, and ages. Much of what we understand about normal sexual function is based on the work done by William Masters and Virginia Johnson in the late 1950s through the 1990s. Masters and Johnson are credited with characterizing the physiologic and biological changes that comprise the sexual response. Later, with the addition of input from Helen Singer Kaplan, desire became incorporated into the model.

One act of sexual intercourse burns 200 calories or is about the equivalent of 30 minutes of jogging.

Sexual intercourse

Sexual contact usually involving coitus or penile vaginal penetration.

Depression

A state of lowered mood usually associated with other disturbances such as sleep issues, loss of or uncontrollable appetite, and loss of life's pleasure. Serious cases may be associated with suicidal thoughts.

Orgasm

The intense pleasurable sensation at the peak of sexual activity or sexual climax usually associated with spasmodic contraction of the pelvic floor muscles. It is often associated with ejaculation, especially in men.

Sensuality, Sexuality, Dysfunction, and Assessment

Following is a description of the phases of human sexual response.

Sexual Desire or Interest

Sexual desire is often characterized as innate hunger or interest in pursuing sexual activity. With respect to female subjects, there is often conflicting data as to normative sexual desire. Some emerging research demonstrates that about one-third of women are based in sexual neutrality, which means that they are responsive to sexual cues from their partners or their environment. (For example, she gets the warm fuzzies at the sight of a special bouquet or box of chocolate.) Another third have a baseline of low to moderate desire on a daily basis, and this can be escalated or diminished depending on the situation or circumstances. The final third may operate more like men, with heightened sense of sexual desire and hunger for the pursuit of sexual activity.

Arousal

The arousal stage of the sexual response cycle is characterized by physical changes in your body. Blood pressure and heart rate become more rapid. Breasts may increase in size and nipples may become erect. The vaginal walls swell, and increased **lubrication** occurs. The clitoris may become swollen, and the inner two thirds of the vagina lengthen. Arousal or excitement is often accompanied with tingling feelings or inner warmth in the genital areas.

Plateau

The plateau is described as the peak of sexual pleasure or plateau right before impending orgasm. Throbbing or feelings of fullness in the pelvis may occur. You may also get a flush on your face, chest, and breasts.

Orgasm

Orgasm is often described as an intense, pleasurable, euphoric, whole-body sensation that is achieved at the peak of sexual

Lubrication

The natural appearance of slippery secretions in the vagina during sexual arousal or the use of artificial lubricants to facilitate sexual activity or intercourse.

stimulation. Rhythmic contraction of the pelvic genital structures (vaginal, anal, and uterine muscles) occurs and an intense feeling of pleasure occurs. Some may have one orgasm and then feel satisfied and complete, whereas others enjoy repetitive multiple orgasms in a row. There are many types of orgasms, including clitoral, vaginal, and uterine orgasms. About a third of women mention that they have rarely or never achieved orgasm from intercourse unless breast and/or clitoral stimulation occurs simultaneously. Some may feel uterine contractions when orgasm occurs; others enjoy the direct pressure of the **cervix** being stimulated. Recently, twin studies have reported that the ease of reaching orgasm may be genetically predetermined and inherited.

Cervix

From the Latin word meaning neck; it is the lower most part of the uterus that protrudes into the vagina.

Resolution

In the resolution phase, heart rate, breathing, and body temperature return to normal or baseline. Blood flows away from the genital and vaginal areas, and you may return to the presexual state of being. Nipples and breasts return to a normal state without arousal. You may feel a sense of euphoria and fatigue.

Originally, sex researchers assumed that women were linear in terms of their progression from one phase of sexual response to another: desire leads to arousal followed by plateau, and then orgasm, and finally resolution. A novel cyclic intimacy-based model developed by prominent sexual health care clinician Dr. Rosemary Basson focuses on a more cyclic experience of female sexual response, where the cycle can be entered at any point. Women experience phases of the sexual response in an overlapping, nonsequential manner that not only incorporates physical but psychological issues as well. An important issue with this model is that sexual desire does not necessarily precede sexual stimulation or arousal. Women may enter sexual activity by being neutral, and then be motivated to enjoy and pursue sexual intimacy to enhance connectedness with their partners. Others may enjoy sex merely for sexual activity.

Sensuality, Sexuality, Dysfunction, and Assessment

Sexual activity creates both positive and negative feelings/ motivations toward subsequent episodes. Receptivity and responsive desire (desire felt after your partner has expressed interest) are key elements in the Basson model. Recent data also suggest that some women follow the original stepwise cascade of the progressive concept of the sexual cycle of desire to arousal to orgasm, whereas others follow the circular pattern as described by Rosemary Basson. Women are unique, and you may ascribe to one model or the other in different circumstances. It is important to understand that sexuality is fluid and that perhaps either model suits you.

It is important to understand that sexuality is fluid.

4. What is normal sexual behavior?

Much of what we understand about normal sexual function is based on the work of Masters and Johnson, who are credited with characterizing the physiologic changes that comprise the sexual response. Normative, or normal, sexual behavior is difficult to define because each unique individual ultimately describes his or her own level of sexual functioning. For example, many couples enjoy twice-weekly sex; others are once-a-weekers. Both may be equally satisfying. On average, most couples have sexual intercourse two to three times a week, but these numbers are definitely affected by a variety of factors such as stress, children, financial pressures, illness, and marital conflicts.

According to a 2003 cover story in *Newsweek* magazine, sexless marriages are on the rise, and it is estimated that 10–15% of couples have sex no more than 10 times per year. It can be difficult to decide what is in fact normal for you as an individual because we are constantly bombarded with sexually voracious *Sex and the City* personalities, Renaissance nudes of ideal nakedness, and movies that depict sex and sensual couples constantly engaged in satisfying sexual activity. In fact, in a 2004 article in the *Journal of Sex Research*, a Canadian study states that 1% of adults are asexual or utterly uninterested in sexual activity. It is also important to understand that normative values of sexual function are defined by the society and culture in which you live. Some traditional cultures are sexually open and expression is permitted, whereas other cultures do not advocate an open expression of sexuality.

Whether you have sex once a week, twice weekly, monthly, or once a year, you and your partner should define normal sexual intimacy as a couple. Deciding on your normative level of sexual interest and activity is an individual journey and often a challenge.

Raye comments:

Normal sexual behavior is hard to define; it is different for everybody. How do you define normal? There are many contributing factors, such as one's upbringing, religion, sexual preferences, ethnicity, culture, and morals. I think everyone has their own definition of what is normal sexual behavior. What I might find normal someone else might find is taboo! What is good for one is bad for another. I also learned that treatment is like ingredients: the healthcare provider can provide a lot of suggestions, and then suggest a recipe, which is perfect for me. I appreciated the individualized approach.

5. What are common sexual complaints?

According to the *Diagnostic and Statistical Manual of Mental Disorders*, 4th edition, there are many categories of female sexual complaints. Classification includes disorders in desire (affecting motivation to engage in sexual activity or thoughts about sexual intimacy), arousal (affecting psychological and physiologic excitation in response to sexual stimulation), orgasm (diminished, delayed, or absent peak intensity of sexual pleasure), and pain (genital or pelvic pain that occurs before, during, or after sexual activity).

Hypoactive sexual desire disorder is the persistent or recurring deficient or absent sexual fantasies and desire for sexual

Libido

Sexual interest or desire.

activity that causes marked distress or interpersonal difficulty. (Most commonly, women say, "My **libido** is low" or "My sexual desire is low." Sexual desire is often called *mojo*, a term that encompasses more than just sexuality and includes an overall *joi de vivre* as well.)

Female sexual arousal disorder is the persistent or recurrent inability to attain or to maintain until completion of sexual activity an adequate amount of genital lubrication or a swelling response of sexual excitement. This disorder causes interpersonal difficulty or marked distress. This disorder has many facets, including subjective arousal disorder (diminished feelings of sexual arousal, excitement, or sexual pleasure; vaginal lubrication does occur), genital arousal disorder (seen in women with nerve damage or estrogen deficiency, where there is minimal vulvar swelling or vaginal lubrication and reduced sexual sensation from caressing the genitals; subjective excitement does occur), and combined arousal disorder (the most common type where both facets of arousal are affected).

Female sexual orgasmic disorders are persistent or recurrent difficulty in, delay in, or absence of attaining orgasm after sufficient sexual stimulation and arousal. These, too, include personal distress or interpersonal difficulty.

Dyspareunia

Pain with sexual intercourse.

Vaginismus

An involuntary tightening of the vaginal muscles when the vagina is penetrated. The action can cause significant distress and pain.

Female sexual pain syndromes include **dyspareunia, vaginismus,** and other pain disorders. Vaginismus is defined as the persistent or recurrent involuntary spasm of the outer third of the vagina that interferes with intercourse. Dyspareunia is a broader term that is often used to describe genital pain associated with interpersonal difficulty. Pain syndromes can be complicated and complex with respect to etiology and treatment plans.

Sexual disorder may be situational (occurs in one situation) or generalized (occurs in all situations), lifelong or acquired, and may have multifactorial components in its etiology.

Raye comments:

The most common sexual complaint is one partner wants sex more than the other person. It is sometimes difficult to be on that same intimate level as your partner and have the same sexual responses and desires as your partner. Most men complain they don't have sex enough, and most women complain that their partner wants to have sex too much. They are also overlapping. After discussion, I realized that I not only had one issue, but that it affected other aspects of my sense of womanhood and sensuality. It all relates together.

6. What is sexual aversion disorder?

According to the American Psychiatric Association's *Diagnostic and Statistical Manual of Mental Disorders*, sexual aversion disorder (SAD) is the active avoidance of or aversion to genital sexual contact with a partner that may cause extreme interpersonal difficulty or distress. The person may be extremely fearful about sexual activity. Psychological factors, severe stress, and need for avoidant behavior as well as past history of emotional and sexual abuse have been implicated in the origin of this disorder.

Patients often implement various avoidant behaviors so that they may limit or circumvent sexual contact. Avoidant behaviors and strategies that have been linked to sexual aversion disorder include excessive traveling for both business and pleasure to avoid sexual partners, alteration of sleep patterns so that sexual activity is unlikely, neglecting personal hygiene, substance abuse, and appearing overtly involved with work commitments, social engagements, or family obligations. Patrick Carnes is a well-known author on the subject and discusses this disorder in his 1998 article "The Case for Sexual Anorexia: An Interim Report on 144 Patients with Sexual Disorders" in *Sexual Addiction and Compulsivity*. He also describes that the person with sexual aversion disorder may partake in extreme efforts to avoid sexual contact,

Antidepressant

The best medication to treat depression and panic attacks. Antidepressants are nonaddictive and may benefit the central nervous system in many ways.

Topical anesthetics

Medication applied to the surface of the body, for example, the skin or mucous membrane, to numb the area.

Estrogen

A steroid hormone produced mainly in the ovaries; the primary female sexual hormone.

Testosterone

A sexual hormone that is produced in the ovaries and adrenal glands that is important in normal sexual functioning. It has been implicated in normal female libido or desire.

Progesterone

A hormone that is secreted by the ovary and placenta (during pregnancy); it is necessary for pregnancy and has been implicated in female sexual function.

including self-mutilation, self-cutting, and gross distortions of bodily image. It is a serious medical and sexual problem that warrants a complex treatment plan that may include medical and psychological intervention.

7. What is persistent genital arousal syndrome?

Persistent genital arousal syndrome is a novel sexual complaint that has recently been discussed within the sexual medicine scientific literature. Sandra Leiblum, noted sexual health-care provider and researcher, is perhaps the world's leading authority and expert on this disorder, which is characterized by persistent burning and throbbing sensations in the pelvic area with intense pressure that is unrelieved by orgasm or self-stimulation. Often women with this syndrome enjoy it, live with it, rarely complain, and have adapted to live with the situation. Sex or self-stimulation is often an attempt for release that is not associated with intimacy or pleasure. There are many case studies in the literature of persistent genital arousal syndrome, some being caused by vein malformation, excessive soy intake, or other anatomic changes. Some women complain of persistent pelvic throbbing after stopping **antidepressant** medications.

There are many possible treatment options that can help women suffering from persistent genital arousal. Sometimes nerve transmissions can be stabilized with such medications as divalproex (Depakote), citalopram hydrobromide (Celexa), gabapentin (Neurontin), clonazepam (Klonopin), imipramine (Tofranil), fluoxetine (Prozac), paroxetine hydrochloride (Paxil), olanzapine (Zyprexa), or even lorazepam (Ativan). Others have tried **topical anesthetics**, including lidocaine; others have used ice applied to the pelvic area. Other proposed treatments include hormonal normalization including normalizing both **estrogen**, **testosterone**, and **progesterone**; surgical excision of irritating lesions/tumors; or embolization of arteries if they are thought to be contributing to this distressing condition.

8. What is involved in sexual activity and love?

Sexual functioning is a complex interplay between biology, physiology, and psychology. Veins, arteries, nerves, genitals, breasts, and nipples as well as an array of hormones, neurotransmitters, and other physical components play important parts in the functioning of sexual activity. The pursuit of coupling has been under investigation for many years, and researchers are always coming up with a variety of answers as to why we love, from whom we seek companionship, and why we are sexual creatures. The trend now is to focus on major histocompatibility complex (MHC), a grouping of genes that controls immunity and influences tissue rejection. Women and men may be attracted genetically to those individuals who can optimize successful conception and procreation. In some recent studies, men and women responded positively to the scent of each other's MHC. Women on birth control, which places them in a state that is chemically similar to pregnancy, are unable to identify and react to their appropriate genetic partners.

When we fall in love, two unique chemicals are released: norepinephrine (NE) and phenyethylamine (PEA). PEA is an amphetamine-like substance that can affect mood and that helps create the wonderful feelings we enjoy when we are in love. Chocolate is also known to contain PEA, which is why many believe chocolate is associated with increased feelings of love and sexual arousal. NE can increase your blood pressure, increase your heart rate, cause palms to sweat, and is thought to help form a connection or help solidify a loving bond to our attraction.

The physiology of the female sexual response includes the pelvic genital organs: **vulva**, **clitoris**, labia majora, labia minora, and the internal pelvic structures of **vagina**, **uterus**, ovaries, and Fallopian tubes. The spinal and central nervous system are also major contributors as are many areas of the brain including the hippocampus, hypothalamus, limbic system, and medial preoptic area. Many neurotransmitters and

Sexual functioning is a complex interplay between biology, physiology, and psychology.

Vulva

The external female genitals also commonly known as the vulvar lips.

Clitoris

The erectile organ in women; the external portion is located at the junction of the labia minora just in front of the vestibule.

Vagina

The part of the female genital tract that connects the uterus to the external vulva. It is 8 to 10 cm in length.

Uterus

The female reproductive organ in which a pregnancy occurs.

Sensuality, Sexuality, Dysfunction, and Assessment

13

Dopamine

A catecholamine that serves as a neurotransmitter and also as a hormone inhibiting the release of prolactin from the anterior portion of the pituitary gland. It is involved in the neurochemistry of sexual function for both men and women.

secondary modulators, neuropeptides such as serotonin, **dopamine**, norepinephrine, epinephrine, opioids, nitric oxide, acetylcholine, and vasoactive intestinal peptides have also been implicated in the response cycle. Some recent research focused on the restoration of serotonin balance as a key factor in female sexual wellness. Sex steroids are essential in the female genital response, and estradiol and testosterone have been clearly implicated in the normative functioning of the female sexual response cycle.

The brain is also a critical area for sex and love. Studies of people's brains who are in love show activity in the ventral tegmental area of the midbrain. Another important area is the nucleus accumbens in the forebrain. Dopamine, serotonin, and oxytocin, which are neurohormones and neuromodulators in the brain, may also influence love, desire, and connectedness. Some new medications in development are centrally acting and act as modulators of serotonin that can create or restore a balance of hormones, thus facilitating a return of sexual desire. Often female sexuality is viewed as an interplay between brain and body.

9. What is the benefit of coupling?

Countless research data show a survival benefit for being coupled or married. In a 2006 study, never-married people were 58% likelier to die in an 8-year period than their married counterparts. Marriage often signals changes: decreased nightclubbing, decreased alcohol consumption, and balanced meals. A Centers for Disease Control and Prevention (CDC) report in 2004 states that married people are less likely to smoke or drink alcohol than single or divorced people are. These changes in lifestyle habits may translate into less cardiovascular disease, cancer, and respiratory problems. Married people also have lowered rates of mental illness, sexual transmitted diseases, and suicide; marriage may help spouses cope with stress.

What are some erotic or erogenous zones? Sexual intimacy not only involves the genitals but other areas of increased sensitivity and sensuality, including the neck, mouth, nipples, underarms, thighs, buttocks, and even the toes. Most women believe that the whole body can be erotic and erogenous. Most healthcare providers in the field of sexual medicine will encourage you and your partner to explore your whole bodies and get accustomed to what feels good for you. Sexual erogenous zones are unique to individuals.

Raye comments:

Coupling has many physical and sexual benefits for most people. We are raised to believe from the beginning that you are to be married and have a lifelong partner. When I was a little, little girl, I wanted the big white wedding and white picket fence and a dog named Spot. It is almost engrained in us that we need to pick a partner to share our lives with. Sharing your life with a partner and sharing intimacy as a couple, I think, is beneficial to both your health and your psychological well-being. I know relationships go through good and bad times, and overall it does take lots of hard work, but the benefits are worth it!

10. What is a sexual history?

A detailed history is critical for correct assessment of female sexual complaints. It is often helpful for you to characterize your complaint in your own words, and your clinician may facilitate this process by being an active listener. For clinicians, understanding the time frame of the complaint is essential. Has it been lifelong? Acquired? Is it present in all situations with all partners or only in selected relationships? Can you attribute the onset of the complaint to a certain event, life change, or trauma?

Your clinician will assess your gynecologic, menstrual, and obstetric history and request a list of medications you take, including any herbs and over-the-counter supplements. Prior surgeries as well as an assessment of ongoing chronic medical illnesses and their timelines and treatments are also required. Your clinician may require a psychosocial, marital, and psychiatric history. Your past medical history, current health status, and that of your partner, as well as an evaluation of your neurologic and endocrine systems can be helpful. Life stressors including financial pressures, employment, and social responsibilities are also critical and can affect sexuality.

Your clinician will attempt to assess and quantify your symptomatology, especially if you experience pain during sex or vaginal dryness. These symptoms can be complex and often encompass urinary or bladder concerns (frequency, urgency, incontinence, and frequent urinary tract infections) as well as vaginal complaints (dryness, painful intercourse, bleeding/spotting, itchiness, pain, pressure, or foul-smelling discharge). Your clinician will assess any symptoms, including stress, anxiety, and depression, and their impact on sexual intimacy or desire. Evaluation of depressive symptoms, domestic abuse, and substance use or abuse is also necessary for a comprehensive detailed evaluation.

Your partner can also be an important source of information, and many women advocate having their partner present at some point during the history. Your healthcare provider should strive to ensure that confidentiality of your health information and continuity between visits is maintained. Also, a positive, safe therapeutic alliance between you and your healthcare provider is critical to successful outcomes.

Sometimes structured, formalized interview scales and checklists can be incorporated into your workup. Do not be concerned or afraid if your healthcare provider asks you to complete some checklists or formal questionnaires. They are helpful in teasing out symptoms and are often used to help diagnose the sexual complaint. Some healthcare providers use checklists and scales for research purposes, so it is always important to ask whether your information will be kept confidential (as it should be). Also, make certain that your name and any other personal identifiers such as address, social security number, or insurance policy number are not on the forms. Some of the more popular screening and assessment tools include the Female Sexual Function Index (FSFI) and the Brief Sexual Symptom Checklist. These questionnaires often are mailed to you in advance or you can complete them in the waiting room. Some healthcare providers make them available on their Web sites for easy downloading and completion.

What is cross-cultural sexuality? Culture plays an important role in our sexual belief system and make-up. Many healthcare providers lack the cultural sensitivity to understand certain cultural issues specific to certain ethnic and racial groups. A healthcare provider lacking cultural awareness may erroneously assume that the poor woman is not interested in sexual function, the quiet Asian woman does not have any concerns regarding intercourse, or the African-American woman is more worried about other healthcare concerns. Some cultures, such as those in West Africa, consider heavier women more attractive than thin ones, whereas some cultures, such as those found in New Guinea, have institutionalized oral sex. Some Islamic cultures practice various forms of **female circumcision**, and polygamy (the practice of having more than one wife), although accepted in some places, is criminalized in the United States. Some cultures permit the viewing of erotic material whereas others find such activities reprehensible.

Understanding your own culture and belief system can help you educate your healthcare provider. The young and the elderly; those who are married, single, divorced, widowed, or partnered; and those of Asian, Hispanic, Middle Eastern, or African-American background are entitled to easy access, assessment, diagnosis, and treatment of sexual healthcare concerns. Sexual wellness and vitality are rights of all women irrespective of their color or social or economic class.

Female circumcision

Any form of ritualized genital cutting or excision or destruction of parts of the female genitalia.

Raye comments:

A sexual history is your complete history pertaining to anything having to do with everything from your sexual past and present. Sexual abuse, partners past, number of sexual partners, pregnancies, STDs [sexually transmitted diseases], complaints, gynecological issues, health, surgeries, illnesses, concerns. I know it is hard to talk about some personal things, but once you find a healthcare provider who is sensitive and caring, he or she can make you feel comfortable. It often takes courage to keep looking for the right healthcare provider when you have had bad experiences, but don't give up.

11. What is a sexual physical examination?

It is often helpful to the clinician to examine your body in the sexual healthcare setting.

It is often helpful to the clinician to examine your body in the sexual healthcare setting. Some of the anatomic structures that your clinician might examine during a sexual physical examination include the following:

Vulva: The external female genitalia not including the breasts. The vulva includes the labia majora and labia minora.

Perineum: The skin between the vagina opening and the anus. The perineum has nerve endings, which, when stimulated, can produce enjoyable sensations during intercourse. The perineum can be injured or traumatized during vaginal childbirth. Delivery with a vacuum or forceps and undergoing an episiotomy (laceration or cutting) can affect the perineum and cause a neuroma, or bundle of sensitive nerve endings, to form and can cause pain during penetration.

Vagina: The vagina is the internal structure that leads to the cervix and uterus. The opening is external and is between 5 and 7 inches long but can expand if needed (childbirth). The walls of the vagina have folds, which also can expand, and the folds have nerve endings, which may be sensitive to touch. The back one-third is more sensitive to pressure. During arousal, there is increased blood flow to the vagina and more natural lubrication is created.

Mons pubis: The mons pubis is a mound of soft flesh that sits directly on the pubic bone. It may be covered by **pubic hair** or groomed according to the woman's interest or desires.

Labia (lips): Labia majora are on the outside, and the labia minora (smaller) are on the inside. In different women, the labia are a variety of shapes, color, and sizes, and no two women are the same. The labia have an abundant nerve supply, and some women experience pleasure when they are touched or caressed.

Clitoris: The clitoris is the female sexual organ that is located where the inner lips meet. The clitoris consists of a rounded area or head (**glans**) and a longer part (shaft) that contains muscular tissue. The tissue of the inner lips covers the shaft of the clitoris (hood). The size and shape is variable among women. There is a high concentration of nerve endings in this area and it is sensitive to direct and indirect touch or pressure. The clitoris is designed for sexual pleasure and this is the organ's only known function. When a woman becomes aroused, the clitoris fills with blood and increases in size. After orgasm, the clitoris returns to its normal size in about 10 minutes. The clitoris can be stimulated through direct or indirect contact. Direct contact with the clitoris by touching, rubbing, finger, vibrator, or tongue can cause intense excitement and sexual pleasure for many women.

Cervix, uterus, Fallopian tubes, and ovaries: These internal female organs are usually assessed with **bimanual vaginal examination**. The cervix is the area that joins the uterus to the vagina; Pap smears assess cells of the cervix. The uterus is a hollow, pear-shaped organ also known as the womb; a fertilized embryo grows in the uterus until delivery. There are two Fallopian tubes, and they are approximately 4 inches long and connect

---

Sensuality, Sexuality, Dysfunction, and Assessment

Pubic hair

Hair that appears on portions of the external genitalia in both sexes at puberty.

Glans

The terminal knob of the penis or clitoris.

Bimanual vaginal examination

Examination of the vagina, cervix, and uterus as well as the other internal pelvic organs with the use of gloved fingers that are inserted into the vagina while the other hand presses on the abdomen.

the ovaries to the uterus; eggs and sperm often join and become fertilized in the Fallopian tubes. The two ovaries produce many female hormones, release an egg monthly, and are located on either side of the uterus.

Dr Laura Bermans recent publication in the *Current Sexual Health Reports* on genital self-image brings forth some interesting results. Women have some misconceptions about their genitals, and some are worried about the shape size or even odor of their genitals. The genital self-image study reiterated that women who have a negative perception of their genitals may have decreased sexual response and sexual satisfaction. The study also found that women with positive genital self-esteem had more sexual desire, less sexual distress, and lowered rates of depression.

Detailed genitopelvic examinations to evaluate and discern urogenital atrophy are paramount and often necessary to rule out underlying pathology or atrophic changes. *Atrophy* is a chronic progressive medical condition that is associated with tissue and organ deterioration and dryness. Urogenital atrophy contributes to atrophic **vaginitis** (inflammation of the vagina) and may lead to sexual complaints in many women. A pelvic examination with careful inspection can reveal a pale, smooth, thinned epithelium (the outermost lining of the vaginal canal) that is extremely friable (fragile). It may even bleed on light touch. The vagina may be dry without lubrication, pale, and may contain petechiae. The vaginal **mucosa** (tissue lining the vaginal canal) might appear flat and blanched instead of the lush pinkish color with associated rugae (ridges and folds) of a healthy vagina. The vaginal tissue will have decreased pliability, elasticity, and stretchability. External genitalia with loss of or sparse pubic hair, introital stenosis (the opening of the vagina becomes tight and narrow, making penetration or sexual intercourse painful), and labial fusion of the labia minora or majora or obliteration may also help pinpoint a differential diagnosis. Evaluation of the vaginal depth as well as the rectal surfaces can be helpful. Palpation of the vagina

Vaginitis
Inflammation of the vagina.

Mucosa
A surface layer of cells or epithelium that is lubricated by the secretions of mucosal glands.

walls can identify points of deep and superficial muscular or pelvic pain, which may require specific physical therapy or trigger point evaluation. The clitoris, clitoral hood, and surrounding structures warrant a comprehensive evaluation. Shrinkage of the clitoral anatomy and introital stenosis are always concerning to the female patient and may signal a decreased estrogen state.

Clinical examination of the tissues for signs of atrophy should include a simple acid/base test with pH paper to assess the vaginal environment. The vaginal pH is typically elevated in those who suffer from vaginitis. Vaginal cytology (cells) can also be used as an adjunct for diagnostic purposes. It is prudent for the clinician to exclude other causes of vaginal complaints such as candidiasis, bacterial vaginitis, and trichomoniasis as well as other sexually transmitted diseases that can interfere with normal vaginal flora. A quick and simple office-based wet mount and whiff test can be performed to exclude any underlying or compounding infectious etiology.

A complete physical examination can also be completed to assess your general health and rule out possible chronic diseases that may affect your sexual response cycle. Thyroid, heart, and lung assessment can also be helpful in the complete physical assessment for sexual complaints.

12. What laboratory test or other radiological evaluations can I expect?

Occasionally, after a complete history and physical examination are done, your healthcare provider may decide that further testing is needed to help confirm the diagnosis. Comprehensive analysis of hormonal profiles (estrogen, testosterone, prolactin, progesterone) is warranted, and the sexual healthcare professional may include a blood work panel as part of the dynamic workup. Some lab tests that may be done include complete blood count; thyroid stimulating hormone; prolactin; adrenal gland precursors such as DHEA and DHEAS; sex steroids such as an estrone, estradiol, progesterone, and testosterone panel including free testosterone; and sex hormone binding globulin. Cholesterol panel and liver function tests may also be included.

Some of the testing must be done after you have fasted briefly, whereas others must be done during specific times of your menstrual cycle to avoid cycle and diurnal variation. Some doctors do measure hormones regularly to monitor progress, whereas others do not measure hormones and do not place much credence in lab tests. This varies from provider to provider.

The importance of many laboratory tests has come into question because there is some concern regarding reliability and normative values for women across the life cycle. Sometimes a pelvic or transvaginal sonogram may be warranted to assess pelvic anatomy and rule out underlying structural pathology. Some other advanced sexual health assessments tools that the sexual medicine specialist may utilize include vulvoscopy (examination of the vulva and surrounding structures with a microscope to rule out underlying vulvar pathology), vaginal photoplethysmography (objective measurement of genital blood flow with a special probe), functional magnetic resonance imaging (used primarily in research settings, where the brain is evaluated), biothesiometry (assessment of pelvic neurologic status), and perineometry (assessment of pelvic floor musculature).

PART TWO

Sexuality and Chronic Illness

What about sexuality and aging?

How does diabetes affect my sex life?

How does cancer affect sexuality?

More . . .

13. What about sexuality and aging?

According to the American Association of Retired Persons (AARP), there are currently more than 33 million Americans over the age of 65. By the year 2011 (just around the corner), the first wave of the young American baby boomers (total of approximately 76 million people) will celebrate their 65th birthday! By 2030, one in five, or 20%, of Americans will be age 65 or older.

Typically, the Centers for Disease Control and Prevention and AARP have in the past focused their efforts and research toward disease management and prevention, health promotion, immunization, and healthy lifestyle management. Little if any effort is directed to maintaining active sexual intimacy as people age.

Although sexual behavior and desires change with aging, the need for intimacy and physical closeness does not dissipate.

Although sexual behavior and desires change with aging, the need for intimacy and physical closeness does not dissipate. Chronic medical illnesses such as high blood pressure, diabetes, cancer, and orthopedic conditions can impair and have significant impact on sexual function and your sexual response cycle. Sometimes all it requires to resolve some issues is some creative thinking, such as adding pillows for comfort, planning sexual activity when you are well rested, or modifying sexual positioning to accommodate minor disabilities.

Many elderly people are on multiple medications, which can affect erectile functioning, orgasm, arousal, and desire in both men and women. These types of issues, too, may sometimes be solved quite easily. The North American Menopause Society conducted a survey of 752 postmenopausal women that showed that half of the women felt happier and more fulfilled between the ages of 50 and 65 years than they did in their 20s, 30s, and 40s. Many women stated that their sexual relationship made it through the menopausal transition unchanged. If their sexual life was satisfying before, then it remained as such after; if it was forced and unpleasurable before, then, unfortunately, it remained the same after **menstruation** stopped.

Menstruation

Vaginal bleeding resulting from endometrial shedding following ovulation when the egg is not fertilized.

The primary key to successful sexuality as you age is to keep the lines of communication open: ask questions, talk, and listen. Although we all want our healthcare providers to be psychic and know exactly what's ailing us, many doctors and nurses are sexually naive—they lack the time, education, and diagnostic skills to identify sexually based disorders. Speak up and be heard. Let your healthcare providers know that sexuality is an important part of your quality of life even if they think that sex is unimportant.

As a patient, you should demand answers and evaluations from your healthcare providers because sexuality, sexual functioning, intimacy, and connectedness are important issues in your quality of life and the human experience. There is no need to continue to suffer. A sexual problem should never be ignored.

For their part, healthcare providers must begin to routinely ask you about your sexual functioning because they cannot treat a problem if they are not aware of it. They must not be afraid to open Pandora's box. They must know of resources in your community and refer you when they are uncomfortable or ill equipped to deal with issues; ignoring a problem will not make it disappear.

A recent article in the July 2007 issue of *Ob. Gyn. News* titled "One Third of Seniors Have Sex Once a Week" discussed the fact that sex remains an important part of their life for people in the age group of 65 to 74 years. The survey of more than 3,000 seniors found that 73% of those interviewed had a spouse or significant other and that of those 73% were sexually active, which was defined as having had at least one sex partner in the previous 12 months. In the oldest group, those aged 75 to 85 years, 23% of men and 24% of women reported having sex once a week or more, and 47% of men and 46% of women reported having less than one sexual episode per month. Dr. Lindau of the Geriatric Section of the Department of Medicine at the University of Chicago stated that the responses of this age group were similar to those reported for participants aged 18 to 59 years. Sexual problems were also common: 62% of men and 70% of women reported one or more sexual complaints, and as a result many avoided sexual intimacy. Forty-eight percent of men and 34% of women had discussed their concerns with their physicians. Self-stimulation, oral sex, and intercourse all occurred as men and women age.

Unfortunately, as a society we tend to shun aging. As we age, many feel pressured to change their appearances to recapture youthfulness and vitality. Cosmetic surgery, hair coloring, and other physical changes occur with increasing frequency in both sexes as people try to recapture the sensual and sexual fountain of youth. Aging and sexual dynamism should not be diametrically opposed—sex with your longstanding partner changes with time, and intimacy and connectedness may often supersede intercourse when medical and or physical barriers prevail. The human spirit, regardless of age, needs and yearns for companionship, touch, and closeness. Close intimate sexual connections are part of humanness and can be experienced and enjoyed until death. There is definitely no age limit to sex and neither should older people be discouraged from making intimate connections.

14. What is the relationship between cardiovascular heart disease and sexual function?

Many women with underlying heart disease or stroke continue to engage in sexual activity well into later life.

Women suffer from heart disease—it is not just a man's disease. Heart disease is, in fact, the number one killer of women. As women age, they are at risk for cardiovascular events, heart attacks, strokes, and other forms of cardiovascular disease. Many women with underlying heart disease or stroke continue to engage in sexual activity well into later life. Sexual concerns are important factors for women with heart disease, and healthcare professionals and cardiologists should be cognizant that these complaints exist.

A recent study examined the prevalence and correlates of sexual functioning in more than 2,700 postmenopausal women with an average age of 67 years, all of whom had heart disease. This large, population-based study found that approximately 40% of the postmenopausal women with coronary artery disease (CAD) continued to engage in sexual activity. It is estimated that at least 65% of them may have had some type of sexual complaint. Sexual problems such as lack of interest, difficulty in arousal or orgasm, and discomfort during sexual activity were found to be common complaints in many women with heart disease.

There are approximately 5 million stroke survivors in the United States. According to the American Stroke Association, four out of five families are affected by stroke. The National Stroke Association Survey claims that one in five stroke survivors suffers detrimental effects to their sex lives. Some practical suggestions can help stroke survivors enhance and continue to experience a fulfilling sexual life: plan sexual intimacy for when fatigue is at a minimum, use pillows liberally for comfort if mobility is an issue, and even explore new body areas to find areas of sensation and sensuality. If talking has become difficult, one suggestion is to try to communicate with touch or massage. Creativity and relaxation are always important as well. If intercourse has become difficult, focus on pleasure and intimacy through other activities including caressing, hugging, and oral and manual stimulation. Lovemaking should focus on pleasure rather than performance.

If you have underlying heart disease or one of its risk factors such as hypertension, diabetes, or obesity, ask your healthcare provider to assess your sexual functioning; your underlying medical illness could be a significant factor in your sexual complaint.

Sexuality and Chronic Illness

15. What is black widow syndrome?

It is well known that throughout the animal kingdom some species of the female black widow spider consume their male partners after they mate and have completed the intimate act. *Black widow syndrome* is a term I use to describe many women I have clinically evaluated who present with reactive lowered libido as a result of their male partners' heart condition. After comprehensive assessment and evaluation, I have found that the origin of their concerns is that they are fearful that sexual activity, sexual excitement, or arousal may induce another cardiovascular event in their partner—in other words, it is safer for them to have no sexual interest because with no interest there is no opportunity for intercourse, and therefore they are safe and can protect their partners from the potential trauma of another heart attack or cardiovascular mishap.

If you suffer from this condition, the treatment for this syndrome includes extensive education of both you and your partner concerning real risks and perceived risks. The incidence of death during intercourse is remarkably low, and most men and women can resume sexual play after a cardiovascular event without any worries. Your cardiovascular surgeon and cardiologist should be able to reassure you and can do some simple, easy tests to ensure good health and sexual satisfaction.

What is a postsex headache? Headaches after sexual activity are often seen as normal, and many men and women suffer from postcoital (after-sex) headaches. Most sexual healthcare professionals are not certain of the cause, but increased blood pressure combined with muscle tension in the head and neck region all may play a role. The headaches can be mild, moderate, or severe and might last from a few minutes to several hours. If you suffer from these types of headaches, see a doctor to ensure that it is nothing more serious going on. Some healthcare providers suggest over-the-counter medications such as anti-inflammatory pain medications prior to sexual activity. Another suggestion is at the first signal of head discomfort, try to change sexual positions, which may influence blood pressure and eliminate some of the muscle tension.

16. How does diabetes affect my sex life?

Diabetes, or sugar imbalance, can affect the sexual function of both men and women. People with diabetes tend to have problems with sexual function earlier in life than people who do not have the disease. How much diabetes affects sexual function may depend on how severe the disease is and how old you are when the disease began. In general, men and women with diabetes are more likely to have episodes of decreased interest in sex. This is especially common when the diabetes is not under good control.

How much diabetes affects sexual function may depend on how severe the disease is and how old you are when the disease began.

Sexual changes are often more subtle in women with diabetes. Diabetes can lead to changes in the architecture of the blood vessels in the vaginal wall, leading to decreased blood flow. This may cause the vagina to be drier than normal, and it may also change the balance between the good and bad bacteria in the vagina, which may lead to repeat genital infections or yeast infections.

Women with uncontrolled diabetes may also experience recurrent yeast infections and, as a result, may experience vaginal pain and discomfort. Pain during intercourse is not infrequent. You may also notice that you are not as easily aroused or that it takes longer to become lubricated and wet. Sometimes medications that you take to control your diabetes can also influence your sexual response cycle, so it is also advisable to seek medical professional care to reassess your medications and see whether they may be contributing to your sexual dysfunction.

Some women with diabetes complain of less sensitivity and less pleasure from touching or stroking during lovemaking. Other women complain of lowered libido, diminished sexual interest, and orgasmic dysfunction. In the author's clinical practice, sexual enhancers, as discussed later in this book, may be helpful if you have difficulty having or achieving an orgasm.

Sexuality and Chronic Illness

Women and men who suffer from diabetes may also experience changes in mood, exhaustion resulting from constant diabetes management, weight gain, guilt over their disease, or even anger about their partner's disease. Your healthcare provider should address all of these other issues as well because they can influence your interest in sexual activity.

Regulation of sugar levels (blood glucose) to within the normal limits is essential to overall health and sexual wellness. Often, the better controlled and treated your diabetes is, the less severe your sexual problems are. An excellent resource is a DVD titled *Sex Intimacy and Diabetes*, a 3-minute informative documentary about intimacy and diabetes; you can obtain this DVD from the Public Health Foundation Learning Resource Center at www.phf.org or 1-877-252-1200.

17. Does fibromyalgia affect my intimate relationships?

According to the National Fibromyalgia Association, women with fibromyalgia often have serious concerns about sexuality and how the disease affects their intimate lives. If you have fibromyalgia, sometimes you might feel too fatigued or in too much pain to seriously think about sexual activity. Sometimes your pain medications can affect sexual interest or libido. Sometimes your energy level dwindles. Often the disease can take over and affect communication between you and your partner as well. Depression and low mood may also confound the situation.

Despite the pain, exhaustion, and side effects from medications, many women with fibromyalgia can enjoy vibrant sexuality. According to Marlie Emmal, author of *Fibromyalgia and Female Sexuality*, sexual activity may actually be good for fibromyalgia pain: "Sexual activity releases natural hormones in the brain and changes hormones in the bloodstream that may affect and decrease pain levels." Carolyn Dodge Adams, the vice president of patient services for the Arthritis Foundation, Southern California Chapter, recommends setting a date with your partner. Try to balance your energy, balance your fatigue, and prepare yourself emotionally. Some women with fibromyalgia can be extra sensitive even to a gentle touch on the skin so that it is uncomfortable; if this is so, it is important to communicate this to your partner.

Warm baths or warming massage oils may be helpful to reduce muscle tension and strain. Massage or physical therapy can elicit relaxation and heighten sexuality. Do not let your muscle pain and fatigue get the better of your intimate life with your partner. Try creative solutions and consult a specialist in sexuality and chronic medical disease.

18. How does thyroid disease affect my sexuality?

Thyroid dysfunction is a common problem for many women, and it should be known that hypothyroidism (underactive thyroid) or **hyperthyroidism** (overactive thyroid) can influence the sexual response cycle in women. Hypothyroidism is a medical condition characterized by abnormally low thyroid hormone production. Some of the common symptoms include fatigue, depression, weight gain, cold intolerance, sleepiness, coarse and dry hair, constipation, muscle cramps, decreased concentration, vague aches and pains, swelling in the legs, decreased concentration, and changes in cholesterol profile.

Hyperthyroidism
Increased thyroid hormone production that can cause symptoms such as anxiety, weight loss, and at times can mimic panic attacks.

Hyperthyroidism is characterized by excessive thyroid hormone production and can have the following symptoms: excessive sweating, heat intolerance, increased bowel movements, tremors/shaking, nervousness, and agitation with changes in heart rate. Some complain of weight loss and fatigue and decreased concentration. Often women can also tell of changes in menstrual flow with decreased monthly bleeding and sometimes irregular intervals between periods.

Sexuality and Chronic Illness

After reviewing the symptoms of each condition, it is clear that some of the symptoms will influence your sexual interest level. Many women with decreased thyroid function suffer from lowered libido. The blood test to assess whether or not your thyroid is functioning properly is one that measures a thyroid-stimulating hormone. Most sexual medicine specialists feel that thyroid dysfunction is an easy test that can account for many organic causes of sexual complaints. In the author's practice in Newport Beach, it has been his experience that close to 10–15% of patients who present with decreased libido have underlying thyroid disorders. Thyroid disease can be easily treated, so it is clear that this should be ruled out as a medical source of lowered libido.

19. Do neuromuscular diseases like multiple sclerosis affect sexuality?

Multiple sclerosis (MS) is a progressive disease of the central nervous system where gradual destruction of the myelin sheath, or coverings of the nerves, occurs. The myelin sheath surrounds and protects neurons, or brain nerve cells, and with their destruction there is a decreased ability of the nerves to carry electrical signals throughout the body, including to the genitals. Women with multiple sclerosis may need more time to get sexually aroused and may often complain of decreased arousal. Some women with this disorder may also have a variety of different patterns of orgasm. These issues are combined with ever present fatigue from increased muscle spasms. Mobility may be difficult and paralysis may inhibit movements.

Loss of bladder control may also preclude feeling at ease because of worry about incontinence or sudden loss of urine. Women may experience changes in sensation in the extremities including the hands, feet, and face, and changed sensation in the breasts and clitoris may make sexual intimacy difficult and a challenge. Often changes in bowel and bladder habits combined with depression may also affect intimate connections.

Women with neuromuscular diseases typically complain of decreased vaginal lubrication and changes in vaginal muscle tone. Clitoral engorgement may also be decreased. Other issues that are related to the nervous system such as bowel problems, spasticity, muscle weakness, body or hand tremor, and changes in attention and concentration can also affect the sexual response cycle. Those with MS may also experience changes in self-esteem and may have mood swings that affect their intimate relationships. Vaginal dryness, pain, muscle spasms, and possible embarrassment over bowel and bladder incontinence can all lead to lowered libido and other sexual complaints with MS.

Many medical interventions can help mitigate the problems for women with MS so that they may enjoy a fulfilling, pleasurable sexual intimate life. Consult with a sexual medicine specialist who is well versed with chronic medical disease to help you and your partner recapture a romantic sensual life.

20. How does cancer affect sexuality?

Sexual concerns are common for women cancer survivors, and many cancer survivors face the additional issues of a changed self-image, fatigue from their cancer therapies, and fear about death and their mortality. Although not life threatening, not having a healthy and active sex life can affect your entire relationship with your spouse or partner, as well as how you feel about yourself. The ramifications of cancer and its treatment can have a serious effect on your sexual satisfaction. Complaints of sexual dysfunction are extremely prevalent in women of all ages and with all cancer types. It is important to ask your healthcare professional for help!

Some complain of having a low libido (hypoactive desire disorder), changes in orgasm, or changes in arousal. Sexual pain disorders such as dyspareunia (pain during intercourse) and vaginismus (reflexive contracture of the pelvic and vaginal muscles) are also prevalent in the female cancer population.

The ramifications of cancer and its treatment can have a serious effect on your sexual satisfaction.

Sexuality and Chronic Illness

33

Nearly one-quarter of those who survived leukemia or Hodgkin's disease have distressing sexual dysfunction.

Sexual dysfunction is often complex and multidimensional, so an individual's treatment regimen may involve several different approaches. Healthy, satisfying sexual functioning and treatment success are affected by a variety of factors including medical illnesses, hormonal levels, relationship concerns, partner availability, underlying psychiatric disorders, general medical well-being, and cultural and religious behaviors.

21. Am I alone or do many cancer survivors experience sexual complaints?

According to 2005 statistics from the American Cancer Society, with increased technological treatments and advancements in diagnostics and therapeutics, an estimated 60% of all cancer survivors will live at least 5 years after their original diagnosis. In recent years, an estimated 11 million people were cancer survivors in the United States; this number is growing exponentially each year. Research shows that sexual complaints are distressing and occur in up to 90% of women who have been diagnosed with cancer. Other studies report the number of women with posttreatment sexual dysfunction as ranging from 30% to 100%.

It is important for cancer survivors to know that they are not alone. If you have some sexual complaints, you can seek help from healthcare professionals who are sensitive to your needs. You may feel embarrassed or ashamed about discussing the issues with your doctors. Maybe you feel that your doctor is ill equipped to deal with sexual issues. Once you have discussed your concerns with your healthcare provider, your physician hopefully should be able to deal with your concerns or be receptive to helping you with these deeply private issues and concerns. Should your doctor be uncomfortable or lack the technical skills to deal with the sexual side effects of cancer treatment effectively, do not get discouraged. Do not give up! Sexuality and intimacy are important quality-of-life concerns and are viewed as critical facets of health, happiness, and feeling connected with both yourself and partner. A sexual problem should never be ignored, and you should seek healthcare professionals who will support you in your quest for survivorship and sexual rehabilitation.

22. What causes sexual problems in the cancer survivor?

A variety of factors can interfere with a woman's sexuality. In addition to her psychological make-up and past experience with intimate relationships and medications, cancer treatments may affect her sexual response cycle and how she as a woman may respond sexually.

A variety of factors can interfere with a woman's sexuality.

The following sections address some cancer treatments that may affect a woman's sexual response.

Surgery

Operative procedures may change the way your body looks, and some procedures may interfere with the nerves in your genital and pelvic area, which are vital to the sexual response cycle. Removal of your reproductive organs, such as **hysterectomy**, or changes in your breasts may affect your self-esteem and influence how you view yourself as a woman. With extensive surgical resection and radical surgery, women often shift their perceptions of their body and femininity. Large tumor resections that involve extensive physical changes, such as bowel removal, may result in functional changes such as ileostomies, colostomies, and ileoconduits that may be perceived as embarrassing or ugly.

Hysterectomy
Surgical removal of the uterus.

Women with breast cancer who have a genetic predisposition for the development of ovarian cancer because of BRCA gene mutations may opt to undergo a prophylactic oophorectomy (risk-reducing **bilateral salpingo-oophorectomy** [RRBSO], or voluntary removal of the ovaries). Women who undergo

Bilateral salpingo-oophorectomy
The surgical term for the removal of both the right and left Fallopian tubes and ovaries.

removal of the ovaries may have negative sexual consequences as well as develop serious concerns about body image and the development of underlying malignancies.

Mastectomy

The removal of the breast.

When breast cancer survivors undergo prophylactic **mastectomy** (removal of the unaffected breast tissue) and reconstruction after breast removal (sometimes with saline/water or silicone implants), sometimes the breast is not acceptable to them. Poor cosmetic results, with scarring and changes in how the breasts look and feel, may affect sexual enjoyment and self-image. Surgical scarring after procedures may interfere with extremity mobility, especially with arm movement. Finding a comfortable sexual position may be difficult or challenging. It has been the author's experience that some breast cancer survivors complain of changes in arm range of motion, where even putting their arm around their partner is a painful experience because of lymph edema and decreased range of motion. These complaints are present in those who have had lymph node dissections and surgical scarring.

Radiation Therapy

Radiation therapy can cause skin changes such as thickening, contractures, or different textures and colors. Other side effects including unexplained fatigue, loss of hair on your head or in the genital area, and gastrointestinal complaints of diarrhea, nausea, and vomiting may all contribute to a lack of sexual interest. Patients and/or their partners may have unfounded concerns about being "radioactive." The truth is that you cannot catch radiation and neither are you considered radioactive if you have undergone radiation treatment.

Vaginal fibrosis with stiffening and hardening of a shortened vaginal vault can be caused by direct radiation to the vaginal area. This can seriously affect a woman's capacity for penetrative intercourse and her genital, pelvic, and clitoral sensitivity during sexual activity. Her sexual sensation or orgasms may be less intense than before, so it may take longer for her to reach the same level of excitement and arousal.

Chemotherapy

Many agents can cause nausea, diarrhea, and membrane irritation and induce premature **menopause**, which can present as hot flashes and vaginal dryness or atrophy. Loss of hair on the head, eyebrows, eyelashes, and hair on the genitals is distressing and affects a female's perception of sexual attractiveness. Chemotherapy-induced early ovarian failure from surgical removal (adjunctive radiation therapy) can cause menopausal symptoms. The symptoms of hot flashes, sleep instability, vaginal dryness, and mood problems also affect desire, sexual interest, and arousal. Vaginal dryness can lead to painful intercourse or penetration.

23. How can maintenance hormonal therapies, which keep my cancer under control, affect my sexual function?

Aromatase inhibitors such as **letrozole** (Femara), exemestane (Aromasin), and anastrozole (Arimidex) and other medications (like **tamoxifen**, a selective estrogen receptor modulator, or SERM) are often used to treat breast cancer and can exacerbate menopausal symptoms. These medications are very effective in controlling disease and preventing it from returning; however, they do have some side effects. Some research has linked SERMs with vaginal dryness and excessive vaginal discharge, vaginal tenderness, changes in orgasm, and diminished libido. But studies examining the effects of tamoxifen on sexual functioning in women are conflicting and inconclusive. The Breast Cancer Prevention Trial states that minor differences in sexual functioning were observed in tamoxifen users versus those not on the medication. In contrast, Mortimer, another researcher, demonstrated no changes in any phase of the sexual response cycle for women on tamoxifen. Some other concerns regarding tamoxifen include increased risk for uterine cancer, stroke, and blood clots.

The aromatase inhibitors block the conversion of testosterone to estrogen and significantly lower the levels of circulating

Menopause

The lack of menstrual cycles for one year; the permanent end of a woman's menstrual cycle.

Sexuality and Chronic Illness

Aromatase inhibitors

Drugs that suppress the body's natural production of estrogen by reducing production of the enzyme aromatase.

Letrozole

An antiestrogen-type of medication in the class of aromatase inhibitors. It inhibits the conversion of testosterone to estrogens.

Tamoxifen

A selective estrogen receptor modulator that is used in the treatment of breast cancer.

estradiol. Although this action is often the objective of breast cancer therapy, it can aggravate menopausal symptoms, cause osteopenia and **osteoporosis**, and affect bone health. These drugs are notorious for causing severe vaginal dryness and can lead to reactive lowered libido. Women often avoid sexual intercourse because of pain and shy away from intimacy to prevent pain. Further scientific trials are needed to specifically address the sexual ramifications of these drugs.

Osteoporosis
A condition characterized by decrease in bone mass and density of the bones resulting in "thinning" of the bones, causing them to become more fragile.

24. What is the relationship between sexuality, terminal illness, and the end of life?

Surprisingly, little is written about and neither is there significant research concerning sexuality and intimacy at the end of life. Many healthcare providers have major difficulty discussing palliative and end-of-life medical care for a variety of reasons. Healthcare providers are taught to preserve and save lives, so death is often misunderstood by doctors as a medical failure. A healthcare provider's personal discomfort with death may be a difficult issue for him or her to overcome.

Sexuality and intimacy are important facets in the death experience.

Sexuality and intimacy are important facets in the death experience. For those who are dying, the touch of a warm hand or the feeling of a caring embrace may be the only connection they have to the world. Intimacy may be a means to say goodbye and maintain emotional closeness with a terminally ill patient or person. Death and dying are often viewed as diametrically opposed to sex, intimacy, vitality, and love. Even when sexual intercourse is technically not feasible, closeness and humanness should be encouraged.

Perhaps the most important consultation I was involved in was when a young woman of 35 called me frantically; she was aware of the fact that she was dying from metastatic breast cancer and her last wish was for her husband to be permitted to be in bed with her and to hold her closely as life ebbed from her body. In a shaky, tired, distressed voice, she begged me to come to the hospital to write an order in her medical chart allowing this to happen. The nurses on the floor were uncomfortable with her husband in the bed with her. The best lesson is that sexuality, intimacy, and connectedness can be enjoyed throughout the life cycle, and it is only our discomfort with intimacy that precludes the human spirit from maintaining its peak of sexual dynamism. Although it may initially be uncomfortable, most dying patients would want closeness and sexual connections up until their passing.

PART THREE

Gynecological Issues and Special Concerns

Can I be sexually active during my pregnancy?

What about menopause and vaginal dryness?

What about sexually transmitted diseases?

More...

25. Can I be sexually active during my pregnancy?

Sexual activity during pregnancy can change throughout the course of the pregnancy, and many women describe increased arousal and desire in the second trimester, especially when the morning sickness and fatigue that they have experienced early on in pregnancy have subsided.

The first phase of pregnancy is sometimes a period of adjustment accompanied by morning sickness, fatigue, and hormonal changes; many women describe feeling decreased sexual interest. Morning sickness and increased sensitivity to smells may also be issues. Sexual thoughts may return in the second trimester. And after the second trimester, as delivery approaches, many couples find sexual positioning challenging; sex may be uncomfortable for the pregnant woman and finding a sexual position that is comfortable may be difficult. Don't give up—side to side and other positions can be used safely. Also, use pillows to help get comfortable.

If you have an uncomplicated pregnancy, there is no reason not to engage in sexual intimacy with your partner.

Some couples fear that sexual intercourse can hurt the unborn baby or even cause preterm delivery, but if you have an uncomplicated pregnancy, there is no reason not to engage in sexual intimacy with your partner. Always consult your physician or obstetrician who is managing your pregnancy, and ask him or her if there are special concerns given your specific pregnancy. Some healthcare professionals advocate abstaining from receptive oral sex for the woman, especially in the last few weeks of pregnancy because cases of air embolus have been reported. But this doesn't mean you cannot be intimate with your partner.

There are many emotional and psychological changes that happen when a couple discovers that they are expecting a child: the fear of the unknown, the desire to have a healthy child, the concerns for providing for family, and the dynamics of a family rather than a couple. Sexual tension can occur throughout the pregnancy, so it is always important to talk about what you are feeling and how it affects your relationship with your partner. Even if sexual intercourse is not possible for some medical or obstetrical reason, there is no reason to stop being intimate and close.

How Mode of Delivery Affects Sexuality

A 2006 issue of the *European Journal of Obstetrics and Gynecology and Reproductive Biology* published the important study of Buhling, Schmidts, and colleagues on the rate of painful intercourse after delivery according to mode of delivery. More than 1,613 women who all gave birth in a tertiary referral center were mailed 16-question questionnaires concerning sexual behavior and painful intercourse. The patients were divided into four groups: (1) uncomplicated spontaneous vaginal delivery, (2) cesarean delivery, (3) episiotomy (a cut in the genital area that helps provide room for delivery) and perineal lacerations, and (4) operative vaginal delivery including vacuum and forceps. Although the response rate was only 41%, almost half of the patients (47%) reported resumption of intercourse at 8 weeks postpartum.

Forty-nine percent of women experienced significant pain on intercourse and significant persistence of pain in the operative delivery group. Although the low response rate may lead to bias, this interesting but small study does suggest some provocative conclusions, including that continued painful intercourse was minimal in those with spontaneous vaginal delivery over those with significant lacerations and vacuum and forceps deliveries. Fortunately, by 90 days post delivery, most women reported resumption of sexual enjoyment.

Discussing sexual health concerns with your healthcare provider after delivery and in the postpartum period is essential. You should not assume that lack of interest and painful intercourse are caused solely by behavior adaptive to new parenthood. Certainly, you are fatigued, up all night feeding the newborn, and attending to his or her needs. However, there

Gynecological Issues and Special Concerns

may be some physical and hormonal issues contributing to your lowered interest or lack of sexual pleasure. Breastfeeding, lactation, and mode of delivery do affect sexual functioning.

26. Can you have sex in the postpartum period?

Technically, the last stage of pregnancy is the postpartum period. Many women report decreased interest and sexual satisfaction in this last stage of pregnancy. Problems associated with fatigue, anemia, and the mode of delivery can contribute to some complaints. Otherwise, there are medical issues that should also be considered. If a woman is breastfeeding, the increase in prolactin (a hormone that helps the woman produce milk for the newborn) can cause *lactational amenorrhea*, or no periods. Many believe that this is an evolutionary response and that there should be no menstrual cycles during the lactation period while the woman is exclusively breastfeeding. This lack of cycling could provide women the opportunity to appropriately space the births of their infants.

In any event, it is important to remember to use birth control during the postpartum period. Many women can have increased vaginal dryness, which may be a causative factor in painful intercourse. Other medical concerns can include thyroid dysfunction and/or problems with healing from your episiotomy or cesarean delivery. Be sure to consult with your healthcare provider and get a comprehensive physical examination. Sometimes hormones and laboratory work may also be necessary.

Transitioning from sexy lingerie teddies to fluffy and cuddly teddy bears if often a challenge for some women and men as well. It is estimated that approximately 70–80% of women who give birth experience some form of "baby blues" or low mood, melancholy, and anxiety after the birth of the baby. This, combined with sleep deprivation, hormonal shifts, and healing from either a vaginal or surgical delivery, can make the postpartum period a difficult time for many women.

Ten to 15% of women may also succumb to postpartum depression, which is a serious medical illness that definitely warrants immediate medical care and treatment.

Men are sometimes consumed with the notion that their love interest is now the mother of their child. Changing from feeling lust to caregiving sometimes is an adjustment that men need time to get used to. The financial burdens of raising children and the pressures to be an excellent father and provider may also be problematic for some men, and these concerns can affect the sexuality of the couple.

Having a child reignites some memories of your own parents. The concerns of being a good parent are also stressors that new parents face on a regular basis. The stress of receiving unsolicited advice from extended family (mother-in-law, father-in-law, and parents) on how best to raise and parent may also increase conflict in the couple. Good, effective communication in and outside the bedroom can be helpful. Sleep when you can, ask for help, and be gracious enough to accept it! Remember that just because you have a child doesn't mean you can't continue to enjoy a sensual and exciting sex life. Plan date nights, hire a sitter, or enlist the help of family and friends. Spend some quality adult time with your lover and partner.

27. What about sex during fertility treatments?

More than 6 million men and women of childbearing age face infertility or the inability to conceive a child naturally. They must see medical specialists called reproductive endocrinologists and undergo many tests to find out what is affecting their ability to get pregnant. Infertility can be a life crisis for a couple.

When you are trying to get pregnant and have strong needs and wants to become a parent, this often leads to stress and disappointment when you must embark on the path of medical infertility interventions. Hormonal injections and timed

More than 6 million men and women of childbearing age face infertility or the inability to conceive a child naturally.

Gynecological Issues and Special Concerns

intercourse and goal setting ("we must have sex . . . to make a baby") can put a lot of stress and strain on a relationship. This stress, coupled with the fact that many procedures are time consuming, costly, and often unsuccessful, can deplete not only your financial resources but your emotional reserves too. Some other forms of conflict may also appear: unfulfilled need or desire for a baby when treatments fail, the feeling that sexual intercourse is work without spontaneity, and withdrawal by your male partner. If a cause of infertility is discovered, often the partner who is responsible feels guilt, shame, and anger.

Hormone therapy

The use of medications to modify or replace hormones that are decreased or absent in the menopause period.

Communication and togetherness are the keys. Sometimes it is important to set limits on the time and amount of treatments you may endure. Others feel that unplanned sex is also needed and the focus on baby making should sometimes be secondary to pleasure.

Yoga

The spiritual practice aiming to unite the consciousness with universal consciousness to achieve harmony.

Communicate and remain unified, eat well, sleep, and seek professional medical counseling if needed. Also, do not be afraid to seek and research other alternatives such as adoption to fulfill your inner desires for parenthood.

Meditation

A complementary medicine practice of concentrated attention toward a single point of reference.

28. What about menopause and vaginal dryness?

With the end of menstrual cycles and the beginning of menopause, a wide variety of menopausal symptoms can occur. Some women complain of increased hot flashes, vaginal dryness, and mood irritability, and others complain of decreased sleep and fatigue. Mood changes and hot flashes are very common and can be contributing factors to lowered interest and sexual problems.

Acupuncture

A traditional Chinese practice of treating a health condition or medical state by inserting needles into the skin at specific points to unblock the flow of energy.

Every woman's experience of menopause is different and unique; no two women experience the same symptoms. Race as well as culture may influence your symptomatology and subjective experience of menopause. Black, Asian, and Caucasian women may have different incidences of complaints with respect to hot flashes and vaginal dryness.

The loss of estrogen can be associated with vaginal dryness and subsequent painful intercourse. The troublesome symptoms of severe and debilitating hot flashes may affect your quality of life and can impair sexual functioning. Be certain to have your hot flashes managed by a healthcare professional. Certainly, a wide variety of methods can be used to control your hot flashes, including hormones (estrogen treatment and estrogen and testosterone for refractory hot flashes). Popular types of **hormone therapy** include conjugated estrogens (Premarin), medroxyprogesterone acetate (Provera), and a combination of both (PremPro) that come in a variety of dosages and have minimal side effects. Another popular regime is estradiol and norethindrone acetate (Ativella). Hot flashes can also be helped by lifestyle changes, including avoidance of caffeine, alcohol, and spicy foods, and by taking some vitamin supplements. Sometimes practical suggestions can help such as using biofeedback, changing clothing or temperature settings, avoiding cigarette smoke, and using a cooling pillow (Chillow) or menopause sleepwear. Paced respirations and controlling the way you breath are also helpful for some women. Sometimes relaxation techniques such as **yoga**, foot reflexology, therapeutic massage, **meditation**, or functionalized **acupuncture** programs can also be helpful with treating both menopausal and sexual complaints. There has been remarkable progress in the field of acupuncture and it is noted to be helpful in the comprehensive management of hot flashes. Sometimes certain medications such as **serotonin reuptake inhibitors** (venlafaxine [Effexor], paroxetine [Paxil]), antihypertensive medications (clonidine, methyl dopa), and a few of the antiepileptics (gabapentin [Neurontin]) have also been shown to be effective in selected patients with hot flashes.

Vaginal dryness is a serious medical issue that many women suffer with in silence. It can lead to decreased vaginal elasticity and poor pliability and stretchability. Many women with severe atrophy or dryness suffer from painful intercourse and may also suffer from frequent urinary tract infections. In recent research, Goldstein and associates address the issues of **vaginal atrophy**, its causes, and its resulting impact on female

The loss of estrogen can be associated with vaginal dryness and subsequent painful intercourse.

Serotonin reuptake inhibitor

A type of antidepressant medication that does not allow serotonin to be taken up again by the neuroreceptors, thereby causing more serotonin to be present in the neuron. These may be used for depression and panic attacks.

Vaginal atrophy

When the vaginal tissues decrease in size, become pale or dry and without lubrication; this is a result of decreased hormonal levels in the woman's body. The tissues can become sensitive and often vaginal atrophy is associated with painful intercourse. Commonly seen in chemical or natural menopause.

Gynecological Issues and Special Concerns

sexual health and function. Vaginal dryness occurs not only in mature women—women who breast feed, those taking certain medications (allergy medications can be big offenders), and those who suffer from a variety of other medical conditions can all experience vaginal dryness. Vaginal dryness can lead to painful intercourse, which then leads to avoidant behavior, resulting in lowered interest—why take part in something if it's painful and uncomfortable?

There are many choices of therapy ranging from vaginal moisturizers and lubricants to minimally absorbed, local vaginal estrogen products such as creams, rings, and tablets that can help restore and revitalize the vaginal mucosal lining (these are discussed later). Nonhormonal vaginal moisturizers or vitamin E can be applied in the vaginal area and can help hydrate the vaginal tissues. Vaginal moisturizers should be used on a regular basis to help hydrate and revitalize the vaginal lining. Lubricants are designed for intercourse. Lubricants, especially those without flavors, colors, and warming additives, can and should be used liberally during intercourse. Avoid using lubricants such as petroleum jelly (Vaseline), extra virgin olive oil, and other household products because they can change the natural balance of your vaginal bacteria and in some women can lead to infections. An excellent lubricant is a water-based gel such as Slippery Stuff, which is glycerin-free. Many women find it helpful to use lubricants prior to intercourse. Some popular lubricants include Astroglide and K-Y Jelly (Johnson and Johnson pharmaceuticals).

29. What is the truth about bioidentical hormones?

Bioidentical hormones have gained popularity and notoriety with many celebrity endorsements, but often the scientific basis for their recommendation is lacking. *Bioidentical* is meant to be interpreted as "biologically identical" or "the same as the body has." Some pharmaceutically produced vaginal cream products, such as estrace cream or Vagifem tablets (NovoNordisk Pharmaceuticals), are bioidentical because they contain

Bioidentical hormones

Hormonal preparations usually of animal or plant origin that have a similar structure to naturally occurring human hormones.

estradiol, which is similar to the estrogen naturally produced in your body. Suzanne Somers's recent book *The Sexy Years* identified bioidentical hormones as safer alternatives to conventional pharamaceutical products that can decrease the effects of aging and promote energy, sexuality, and youthful appearance among other claims. Mass marketing and media have at times, unfortunately, duped women into believing that compounded estrogen products such as Bi-est (80% estriol + 20% estradiol) and Tri-est (80% estriol + 10% estradiol + 10% estrone) are safer hormones and have no health risks or adverse problems, such as breast cancer risks.

Most compounded products are not subjected to rigorous clinical testing for consistency, purity, safety, or efficacy. If you use bioidentical compounded products, it is important for you to know that they are subject to the same risks as conventional pharmaceutical hormonal therapy. A detailed review of more than 40 years of medical research on estriol, however, found no evidence that it is medically safer or breast protective. In addition, there is no scientific evidence to support the use of salivary gland hormone testing in women; there is no evidence that these values have any biological meaningfulness. There is no relationship between salivary levels and serum or blood levels, and there is large variability in salivary hormones, which are dependent on diet, time of the day, specific hormone tested, and other variables.

Both the North American Menopause Society (www.menopause.org) and the American College of Obstetricians and Gynecologists (www.acog.org) have come out with strongly worded positions statements against recommended compounded hormonal products. The **Food and Drug Administration** also has stated that estriol is a misbranded drug because of unsubstantiated claims of efficacy, superiority, and bioidentity. Of interest, estriol is presently classed as an unapproved new drug under Section 505 of the Federal Food, Drug, and Cosmetic Act. It is important to ask questions about bioidentical hormones and their consistency and purity.

Food and Drug Administration (FDA)

Federal agency that protects public health by regulating the safety and efficacy of food, medical products, biotechnology, and cosmetics. No drug or device can be sold on the market unless it has undergone vigorous scientific testing and passed the strict regulations of the FDA.

There are risks involved in all hormonal products and compounded products are not immune to serious health concerns.

30. How do fibroid tumors, tubal ligation, and endometriosis affect sexual function?

Fibroid

A benign tumor arising from smooth muscle cells of the uterus.

Fibroids are benign (not cancerous) tumors that originate from smooth muscle cells of the uterine muscle. They can be within the uterine wall, on a stalk (pedunculated), protrude into the abdominal cavity, or be on the inside and affect the uterine cavity where a baby grows. Studies on fibroids, or uterine myomas, and sexual function are often conflicting; some indicate that women with fibroids have more sexual complaints, more painful intercourse, and lowered sexual interest, whereas other studies do not support these findings.

You may experience many symptoms from fibroids, including abnormal uterine bleeding, pressure, chronic pelvic pain, and gastrointestinal symptoms. All of these symptoms can influence your sexual interest. About 20–40% of all women have fibroids and are experiencing some sexual complaints. It is best to get a comprehensive evaluation by a gynecologist or sexual medicine specialist. If your pain can be linked to your fibroids, sometimes surgical intervention can be helpful, but it depends on where the fibroids are located. You may need a pelvic ultrasound so that you and your healthcare provider can get a clearer picture of where the fibroids are located. Fibroids can be removed with hysteroscopic techniques (where a small tube is inserted into the uterus through which the provider can operate using small instruments and thereby remove the fibroids), with laproscopic techniques that are minimally invasive, or by making an abdominal incision.

Where the fibroid is located can also possibly affect sexual pain. If the fibroid is large and affecting other pelvic or genital structures, it can be uncomfortable during penetration. If the fibroid is small, it is likely that it will not affect sexual function. If you have fibroids and think they are contributing to your disinterest in sexuality or are playing a role in sexual pain, seek medical attention and get a transvaginal ultrasound to properly assess position, size, and number of fibroids. A variety of treatment options is available including less aggressive medical treatment such as medications like nonsteroidal anti-inflammatories and gonadotropin-releasing hormone (GnRH) agonists, as well as surgical interventions.

Tubal ligation, or permanent irreversible sterilization through surgical technique, has not been extensively studied when it comes to sexual function. It is unlikely to change sexual interest or pleasure, and the majority of women who undergo this procedure experience positive sexual effects as a result of the freedom from fear of unwanted pregnancy. Most scientific studies on tubal ligation conducted in the United States and Europe report no effects on sexual intercourse.

It is estimated that up to 10 million women suffer from endometriosis, a condition that occurs when the normal lining of the uterus has migrated to other areas of the pelvic region. It is associated with severe chronic pain and also painful intercourse on deep penetration. Other complications can include abnormal bleeding and severe pain. Although the cause of endometriosis is not specifically known, there are multiple treatment options including medications (anti-inflammatory medications such as ibuprofen [Advil or Motrin] or oral contraceptive pills). Stronger medications such as narcotics can influence the sexual response cycle. Surgical ablation or removal of the endometriosis may be helpful. Some women do eventually need a hysterectomy, or removal of the uterus, ovaries, and Fallopian tubes. Endometriosis has been linked to sexual pain and painful intercourse, so if you are experiencing sexual pain, it may be a good idea to be assessed for this gynecological syndrome.

Gynecological Issues and Special Concerns

31. How can oral contraceptives affect sexuality?

Perhaps the most controversial topic of debate that has been discussed in the field of sexual medicine is that of oral contraceptive and its influence on female sexual function. Again, the data are conflicting with respect to research and hormones. The opponents of oral contraceptive pills tout the increased levels of a protein called sex hormone binding globulin (SHBG) as a result of the oral estrogen component of the oral pills. This increase in SHBG results in a lowered free testosterone level, which many have translated into a lowered sexual interest. Although androgens including testosterone are linked to sexuality and female sexual interest, the extent to which these hormones play in female sensuality and sexuality remains to be elucidated.

Interestingly, many other studies do not support the claim of changes in sexual function with the use of oral contraceptive pills. Many report neutral effects on sexual function given their chemical and hormonal make-up, like Loestrin 24, by Warner Chicott. This pill has a shorter pill-free interval, so women who suffer from premenstrual syndrome-like symptoms have increased symptomatic relief and henceforth increased sexual interest. The same can be said for Yaz (Bayer Pharmaceuticals); since it is often prescribed for acne, this may help eliminate social isolation in the acne sufferers who may experience a boost in sexual self esteem on the medication. There are recent concerns regarding this medication and overstated efficacy as well as potential problems with increased potassium. Donnerstein, a noted sexual medicine specialist in Australia, published research indicating that women's sexual function is more closely linked to their partners health than to their androgen levels.

Some potential benefits of birth control pills include lessened premenstrual syndrome, less bleeding, decreased anemia, and stabilization of pain from endometriosis. If these symptoms contribute to your sexual complaints, minimizing them may be associated with renewed interest in sexuality. Other studies support the notion that women who are on birth control pills have an increased sexual freedom—freedom from fear of unintended pregnancy is often liberating for the sensual woman.

Before automatically jumping to conclusions and assuming that oral contraceptives are the answer to your sexual complaints, be certain to undergo a comprehensive assessment, which should include a history, physical examination, and laboratory work. Although the pills may be a minor contributor to solutions, it is wise to seek professional care from your sexual healthcare specialist.

If, in your case, there are issues with oral contraceptive pills, safe alternatives for effective contraception include the intrauterine device (IUD), implantable contraception that releases hormones, abstinence, condoms (male and female), and permanent, irreversible sterilization. These can be effective methods of contraception with varying failure rates.

Raye comments:

Oral contraception is not liked by everyone. Some women cannot tolerate it for different reasons; however, I personally think it does have many positive influences on sexuality. With birth control comes more sexual freedom. With more sexual freedom you may experience more interest in sex as well as an increase in your overall libido. The Pill can be positive because it decreases cramps and blood flow, and most important it protects you from pregnancy. Not having to worry about that alone might make you more sexual.

32. What is vulvodynia?

Vulvodynia is a condition characterized by a multitude of vaginal and vulvar complaints that can include burning, itchiness, and painful intercourse. Although there are many working diagnoses of the etiologic causes of this type of vulvar pain, none is proven to be the definitive answer. Vulvodynia is associated with sexual pain and discomfort, and many women

Vulvodynia is a condition characterized by a multitude of vaginal and vulvar complaints that can include burning, itchiness, and painful intercourse.

with this condition have stopped having intercourse. Many women suffer from this condition for many years until the definitive diagnosis is made, and many go unrecognized or untreated for many years.

If you have vulvar complaints, seek medical care from a specialist. Along with a complete history and physical examination, some of the following tests may be done to form a diagnosis: cotton swab test, vulvoscopy, measurement of vaginal pH secretions, and genital cultures to exclude sexually transmitted diseases like gonorrhea and **Chlamydia infection**. A wet mount or slide preparation of the vaginal discharge will sometimes be made to see if there are other infectious processes going on as well. Vulvodynia may be associated with interstitial cystitis, so it is also important to have a complete genitourinary assessment.

Some doctors also advocate a comprehensive hormonal panel as well as a **biopsy**. The National Vulvodynia Association (www.nva.org) is the best resource for those suffering from vulvodynia. Some of the treatments have included strict vulvar care with avoidance of allergens, and application of cold compressors and topical numbing medication 20 minutes before **coitus**. Hormones such as estradiol alone or combined with testosterone in methylcellulose/petrolatum applied to the vestibule may also be helpful. Topical estrogen creams have also been used with moderate success; they are safe and effective treatments for this condition. Biofeedback and physical therapy have also been used with some success. Acupuncture, the traditional Chinese medicine technique of needle insertion to promote increased chi and bodily energy, has also been tried to help with chronic pain and discomfort. Other medications taken orally or applied topically that have also been used include tricyclic antidepressants, gabapentin, and intralesion interferon. Some more experimental methods include low-oxalate diet with calcium citrate supplementation, topical capsaicin, suppressive antifungal therapy, and topical lidocaine every 6 hours. Some researchers advocate keeping a food diary; some women have linked their symptoms to

Chlamydia infection

A sexually transmitted disease caused by the infection with the bacterium *Chlamydia trachomatis*.

Biopsy

A surgical procedure that involves obtaining a tissue specimen from the body for laboratory testing to determine a more precise diagnosis

Coitus

Latin word for the penetration of the vagina with a penis.

specific foods such as blueberries, strawberries, and spicy foods. Surgery to remove the skin that is causing the burning or other symptoms should be reserved for refractory cases, and many are not completely helped by such vestibulectomies.

According to the National Vulvodynia Association, many women have very sensitive vulvar areas that can be easily irritated and lead to painful irritative symptoms including painful intercourse. Following is a list of some practical suggestions to help maintain vulvar health. The list is from the NVA.org handbook:

- Wear all-white cotton underwear.
- Do not wear pantyhose (wear thigh-high or knee-high hose instead).
- Wear loose-fitting pants or skirts.
- Remove wet bathing suits and exercise clothing promptly.
- Use dermatologically approved detergent such as Purex or Clear.
- Limit fabric softener.
- Double-rinse underwear and any other clothing that comes into contact with the vulva.
- Use soft, white, unscented toilet paper.
- Use lukewarm or cool sitz baths to relieve burning and irritation.
- Avoid getting shampoo on the vulvar area. Do not use bubble bath, feminine hygiene products, or any perfumed creams or soaps.
- Rinse the vulva with water after urination.
- Urinate before the bladder is full.
- Use 100% cotton menstrual pads and tampons.
- Be careful of contraceptive creams or spermicides. Read labels. Often many products contain irritants or allergens that can affect an already sensitive vulvar area.

33. What is lesbian sexuality?

Lesbian sexuality and the sexual health needs of other minorities have often been neglected in the medical publications and in the lay press. Approximately 3–5% of the female population are self-identified lesbians who enjoy same-sex relationships with partners. Many are in long-term committed relationships that share social, financial, and child-rearing responsibilities. Lesbians engage in a wide variety of sexual behavior from intimate touching and kissing to mutual penetration, and some may use sexual accessories such as strap-on paraphernalia. Sharing of sexual toys and oral sex may also be a part of the sexual repertoire.

According to the Lesbian Health Fund founder Kate O'Hanlan, who is also the former president of the Gay and Lesbian Medical Association, lesbians have many healthcare concerns that should be discussed with their healthcare providers including breast cancer (lesbians have many risk factors, and for a wide variety of health reasons many over the age of 40 do not get regular **mammograms**, do not do breast examinations, and do not receive clinical breast examinations), depression, and anxiety.

Mammogram

A special X-ray of the breast tissue that can be used as a screening tool for breast cancer.

Other issues related to psychiatric illnesses are important possibly resulting from chronic stress from homophobia, stress from family, and unfriendly work and social environments. Substance abuse and excessive tobacco and alcohol use are also important issues to be addressed. Gynecologic and cardiovascular health care are critical because many lesbians are overweight, smoke, and do not get screened for diabetes, high cholesterol, or blood pressure. Fitness health issues should also be addressed because obesity may also be more common in the lesbian population. Domestic violence and osteoporosis are other health concerns of lesbian patients and should be discussed during the annual gynecologic examination.

Some illnesses or surgical procedures that affect the breasts may also adversely affect the sexual pleasure of lesbians who focus on breast caressing and stimulation for a large part of their sexual arousal. Those with breast cancer and surgical alteration or removal of the erotic organ may feel distressed and saddened by the loss of this sexual organ. Clitoral arousal and stimulation may also be affected by medications that blunt arousal (depressive medications). *Lesbian bed death* is a term invented by sex researcher Pepper Schwartz to describe the supposedly inevitable diminishment of sexual passion in long-term lesbian relationships. The term is sometimes used to refer to diminished sexual activity in any long-term relationship.

34. How common is same-sex attraction?

Gay men and lesbian women are becoming more visible in today's society. Rosie O'Donnell, Ellen DeGeneres, Nate Berkus, and novelist Armistead Maupin have increased awareness of homosexuality to the lay public. Still, the United States may be decades behind the world in granting equality to homosexuals, ending discrimination, and promoting safe health policy, financial protection, and penalties for hate crimes based upon sexual orientation. Canada, Holland, and many other progressive countries have embraced all their constituents and have accepted gay unions—many have gone as far as to endorse the freedoms of same-sex couples with laws to protect their unions and their families. Many countries support same-sex marriage.

Gay and lesbian men and women raise families, work, pay bills (and enormous tax bills partly because of the lack of tax protections that heterosexual couples enjoy), prepare and clean up meals, attend the PTA meetings, and enjoy the humdrum life of parenthood and couplehood. The emerging trend in medical science is that sexual orientation is not environmentally determined but may be determined by a complex interplay between genetic make-up, hormonal environment, and other complicated conditions of development.

Same-sex relationships have been around since the beginning of time and are even prevalent in nature and in the wild. Consider the pink flamingo! In Bristol, England, a pink flamingo named Fernando and his partner Carlos has been living in same-sex wedded fowl bliss in the wild fowl animal park. Fernando and Carlos have even adopted an abandoned

Still, the United States may be decades behind the world in granting equality to homosexuals, ending discrimination, and promoting safe health policy, financial protection, and penalties for hate crimes based upon sexual orientation.

Gynecological Issues and Special Concerns

57

chick. A park spokeswoman states that when there are not enough female flamingos or when opposite-sex birds do not hit it off, males pair-bond together. The Flamingo Wildlife Habitat in the Las Vegas Hilton also houses a gay couple of flamingos named Bubblegum and Pink Floyd. In New York City, a pair of male penguins has bonded and is raising a chick—they were the inspiration for the famous and well-received children's book titled *And Tango Makes Three!* At the San Francisco Zoo, a tour will show geese, sea gulls, penguins, lions, and some hoofed animals in homosexual relationships. The zoo relates a story of a pair of female geese that have been happily married for many years. Other examples abound: a pair of gay vultures at the Jerusalem Zoo have shown the world just how talented and caring gay adoptive parents are when an Israeli zoologist Shmuel Yidov placed a day-old vulture chick that had been hatched in an incubator in with the pair. Fooled, the pair took turns sitting on it and warming it until it hatched again. Bisexuality is the norm among male chimps, and a male chimp can form a long-term partnership with another male that often includes sex. Rats, rabbits, and cats also display same-sex relationships. Perhaps we have more to learn from the animal kingdom.

35. What about sexually transmitted diseases?

With the diagnosis of a sexually transmitted disease (STD) such as Chlamydia infection, trichomoniasis, gonorrhea, pubic lice, genital herpes, human immunodeficiency virus, hepatitis, and syphilis comes much fear and anxiety. If you have an STD, not only are you concerned about the immediate health impact of the disease but also its potential to affect future childbearing capabilities and future sexual function.

Some women develop a phobia of sexual function as a result of contracting a disease from a partner. Others struggle with the concept of disclosure: when should you tell a potential partner of your history of herpes infection or warts (human papillomavirus) infection, for example? Still others who are unable to cope turn to support groups and seek out partners who also have the infection. Many tell heart-wrenching stories of disclosure with subsequent rejection from a once-believed understanding partner.

There is no clear-cut answer as to when it is appropriate to disclose personal information about a past infection; on your very first date or just as clothes are being taken off before the first sexual interlude may not be the best time, however. Disclosure is a personal decision and only you know if and when it is appropriate to discuss these issues.

After experiencing a sexually transmitted disease, many women must decide whether to introduce safer sex practices into a relationship. Women will often insist on condom use, and men often cite condom phobia or other concerns such as condoms affecting potency, erectile vigor, and sensitivity/allergy concerns. This may impart additional conflict on an already-strained relationship. Effective communication is the key. Understanding key issues and the medical basis for sexual diseases is important. If sexually transmitted diseases are contributing to your sexual complaints, discuss your concerns with your healthcare provider or sexual medicine specialist.

Raye comments:

*Sexually transmitted diseases are definitely on the rise. I remember just about 10 years ago when I was in high school, sexually transmitted diseases were not what we were being educated or warned about; it was pregnancy. For single women in this day and age it is so frightening. Sex is scary! Protecting yourself is not only a must, but so is **monogamy** and having a trusting relationship with anyone you are sexually active with. What scares me the most is not even condoms are 100%—you really need intimacy and a strong emotional bond with your partner!*

If sexually transmitted diseases are contributing to your sexual complaints, discuss your concerns with your healthcare provider or sexual medicine specialist.

Monogamy

Sexually exclusive couple who do not have sexual relations with other people outside their relationship.

36. I have had a hysterectomy! How can I get help?

A total hysterectomy, which is the surgical removal of the uterus, ovaries, and cervix, is the most common nonobstetrical surgical procedure performed in the United States. There is considerable interest concerning the sexual ramifications and implications after this very common operative procedure. Many feel that the cervix is necessary for excellent sexual satisfaction, and some researchers are now asking a hard question: Should women opt for a supracervical hysterectomy, which leaves the cervix in place to better preserve sexual function? Clearly, some women do have sensation in their cervices and feel them when they have penetrative intercourse; in such cases, a complete and frank discussion with your healthcare provider and surgeon is warranted. A few women describe orgasmic changes after removal of the cervix and uterus.

However, many well-designed medical research studies and published studies fail to provide a solid link between total hysterectomy with cervix removal and sexual complaints. Many studies do show the opposite and even demonstrate an improved sex life after the organs are removed. No study is perfect and obviously many women undergo hysterectomy for debilitating symptoms like severe pelvic pain and enlarged fibroids that are affecting bowel or bladder health. When the hysterectomy is performed and symptoms have resolved, and patients are suffering less, this may translate into better sexual activity.

If you are planning to undergo a hysterectomy, discuss your concerns regarding sexual activity with your healthcare provider before the procedure. Ask questions and have them answered. Seek out healthcare professionals who will listen to your concerns about sexuality and quality of life.

37. What will happen if I have my ovaries removed?

The ovaries produce hormones, and when you are cycling the ovaries produce an egg each month that can be fertilized. The ovaries are also subject to a variety of diseases such as cysts and cancer. Many women fear ovarian cancer. It is a serious, deadly disease that does not have specific early symptoms, and by the time there are obvious symptoms the disease has usually progressed to an advanced stage. Although the medical profession has made strides in treating ovarian cancer, the survival rate is not substantial with advanced disease and recurrence is very probable. Some women have taken the serious step to have their ovaries removed after childbearing, and others who have genetic predispositions to developing ovarian cancer also have opted for risk-reducing removal of the ovaries.

The ovaries are also subject to a variety of diseases such as cysts and cancer.

Even after menstrual periods have stopped, the ovaries have been known to produce testosterone. Some researchers are now investigating the postmenopausal ovary and its endocrine functions. If you are not menopausal and you suddenly remove your ovaries, you will experience sudden menopause—not only hot flashes and vaginal dryness, but emerging data also suggest cardiovascular, bone, sexuality, and even some memory issues.

Robson and associates at Memorial Sloan Kettering Cancer Center published an article in *Gynecology Oncology* titled "Quality of Life in Women at Risk for Ovarian Cancer Who Have Undergone Risk Reducing Oophorectomy." This is the largest study that examined quality-of-life concerns for a subset of women who underwent a risk-reducing bilateral salpingo oophorectomy (RRBSO) as part of a risk reduction strategy to decrease ovarian cancer risk. Questionnaires including a sexual function questionnaire were completed at a mean of 23.8 months after surgery. Estrogen deprivation symptoms such as vaginal dryness, painful intercourse, and dyspareunia continued to be bothersome. Patients continued

Gynecological Issues and Special Concerns

to have considerable distress about sexuality and even worried about developing ovarian cancer in spite of the risk-reducing surgery. RRBSO is a beneficial intervention that reduces ovarian cancer risk; however, from this provocative study, you can see that this simple surgical intervention has serious long-lasting side effects that cause patients personal distress. It has a profound impact on quality of life concerns, especially sexual function. The surgery may not even lessen the patients' anxiety for developing ovarian cancer. This study along with others in the medical literature reiterate the long-held belief that we must strongly consider lasting ramifications from any surgical intervention. Have a frank discussion with your surgeon about side effects and possible sexual side effects from the surgery.

PART FOUR

Pearls for Treating Sexual Complaints

How do chronic systemic illnesses affect sexuality?

How do medications affect sexuality? Can anything be done if I am taking a medication that is affecting my sexuality?

What is Tantra and how can it help sexual intimacy?

More . . .

The treatment of female sexual complaints is complex and involves the combined approach of treating the woman's medical issues as well as assessing and treating her sexual psychological issues. There is no widely accepted paradigm and no set preconceived correct treatment pattern that will help all women. Women are unique in their experience of sexual problems, and thus their treatment plan should be dynamic, unique, and incorporate many facets tailored to individual and personal needs and wants. There is no cookbook for success. Discussed here are a variety of therapeutic options that women suffering from sexual problems may try on their own or with the assistance of sexual medicine specialists. Many interventions have been proven effective in a variety of clinical scenarios. Many have emerging data to support their use. As a person who is affected by changes in sexuality, you may pick and choose some interventions to help effectively treat your sexual complaints.

38. How do chronic systemic illnesses affect sexuality?

Patients with sexual complaints may have other underlying medical conditions and illnesses that directly affect their sexual health and sexual response cycles.

Patients with sexual complaints may have other underlying medical conditions and illnesses that directly affect their sexual health and sexual response cycles. Evaluation and treatment of chronic illnesses, such as uncontrolled hypertension, hypercholesterolemia, and/or an underlying thyroid dysfunction, can be simple to identify and treat. For example, arthritis may affect your mobility and make finding comfortable sexual positions a challenge. Uncontrolled diabetes may influence veins, arteries, and nerves in the genital pelvic region, which may affect blood flow and directly affect excitement (vasocongestion and pelvic engorgement). Underlying genital infections and abnormal discharge resulting from infections like *Candida* (yeast), bacterial vaginosis, and trichomoniasis should also be assessed and treated if present. Sometimes oral medication is best for treatment of infections because the vaginal tissues are delicate and easily irritated.

It is critical to optimize your overall health and treat medical conditions. General health maintenance should never be ignored. Often, sexual specialists include screening physical examinations to rule out underlying diseases or infections and may perform laboratory blood work such as a complete blood profile, complete lipid profile, glucose screening, and prolactin levels. Estrogen, testosterone, and progesterone as well as other hormonal profiles are typically measured, too. Sometimes if you are suffering pelvic spasms or heightened muscle tone, you may be referred to a special pelvic floor physical therapist who can teach you to perform muscle relaxation exercises in the pelvic floor to help reduce pain and muscle tension. A series of pelvic floor sessions with a specially trained physical therapist may also be helpful if you suffer from vulvodynia or vaginismus. The pelvic floor physical therapy specialist is specifically trained in physical therapy that deals with the pelvic floor muscles, and you should ensure the therapist has adequate training and certification before embarking on a treatment plan with him or her.

In the acute crisis of cancer care, sometimes preexisting medical illnesses can be neglected. So, treating any underlying chronic medical illnesses not only improves your general physical and mental well-being, but may also improve your sexuality. Chronic discomfort or pain can influence your sexual response and limit your interest in and enjoyment of sexual activity. When pain is at low level and fatigue minimal, sexual expression should be encouraged. Techniques such as warm soaks and physical therapy help loosen tense muscles. Guided imagery, meditation, deep-muscle relaxation, and avoidance of exhaustion are options that should be explored. You can consult specifically trained pain management specialists to adjust or reduce opioid regimens, add adjunctive or alternative analgesics, and modify existing dosing schedules, which may lessen fatigue while maintaining sufficient pain relief.

Pearls for Treating Sexual Complaints

39. How do medications affect sexuality? Can anything be done if I am taking a medication that is affecting my sexuality?

Many classes of drugs can affect the female sexual response cycle and cause sexual problems. Many antidepressants and antihypertensive medications can affect and alter female sexual desire, arousal, and orgasm. Ask your physician specifically to check pharmacologic guides and guidebooks to identify potential offending agents and discuss substituting another drug, one with less sexual side effects. Also, sexual pharmacology textbooks are available for quick and easy reference and you can check the Internet.

Some of the common medications that can affect sexual response cycle include antihistamines for hay fever or seasonal allergies, blood pressure medications, tranquilizers, and some of the common ulcer medications. Many women take daily antiallergy medications for hay fever or other seasonal allergies, and these medications dry out mucosal membranes and will also affect vaginal health and wetness. Consider limiting them and use a good lubricant as well. Antidepressants are commonly prescribed to women for mood issues and depression, and some women are on the selective serotonin reuptake inhibitors (SSRIs). These medications may affect and delay orgasm in both men and women. Commonly prescribed SSRIs include fluoxetine (Prozac), paroxetine (Paxil), and sertraline (Zoloft).

If you are on a medication and can positively link your origin of sexual problems to beginning this medication, discuss the situation with the prescribing healthcare provider.

If you are on a medication and can positively link your origin of sexual problems to beginning this medication, discuss the situation with the prescribing healthcare provider—do not automatically stop or wean down a medication to lessen the sexual side effects. Discuss alternative medications, drug holidays, or other solutions with your doctor or provider.

Some young women on birth control pills complain of sexual issues. The biochemistry in these tablets may decrease free bioavailable testosterone, which *may* be linked to lowered sexual desire and interest. Simply switching these women to an alternative form of contraception may improve sexual functioning. Others do not mention any complaints while on birth control pills, and the studies are confusing at best. Discussion of contraceptive options with your provider is essential.

The medical treatment of sexual dysfunction often includes changing medication regimens, altering dosing and/or time intervals, or switching to a new drug. Never abruptly stop any prescribed medication without first consulting with your prescribing physician. There may be a good alterative or one that causes fewer or less intense side effects.

You may be able to remain on your medications even if they are affecting your sexual function. Specific anecdotes may be available. New, exciting research was recently published that shows that women who suffer from sexual dysfunction as a result of their antidepressant medications (like serotonin reuptake inhibitors) may benefit from a trial of phosphodiesterase inhibitor medications (**sildenafil**/Viagra (Pfizer Inc.), tadalafil/Cialis (Eli-Lilly and Company), vardenafil/Levitra (GlaxoSmith Kline/Schering-Plough)). These drugs, although primarily FDA approved for men, are now moving to the forefront in the management of some female sexual complaints.

Sildenafil

A phosphodiesterase inhibitor that is used in the treatment of male erectile dysfunction. New data suggest this class of medication can sometimes be used for the treatment of serotonin reuptake inhibitor–induced female sexual problems.

40. What are structured sexual exercises and what is behavioral modification? How do these help treat sexual complaints?

Patients with sexual complaints are always encouraged to make lifestyle modifications that will enhance and improve quality of life. At the Southern California Center for Sexual Health and Survivorship Medicine, we often use a holistic approach and stress diet, exercise, and lifestyle changes to promote sexual health and wellness. A well-balanced nutritious diet with appropriate caloric intake and adherence to the Food Pyramid is important. Increased fruits and vegetable as well as a diet rich in antioxidants is also encouraged. Diet combined with an active aerobic exercise plan is vital. A vigorous exercise plan can increase brain endorphins, which are natural pain killers, and also release a variety of mood-enhancing neurohormones. Stopping the use of tobacco and illicit drugs is important. Minimizing alcohol consumption is also encouraged. If fatigue or tiredness is a problem, we encourage you to take frequent naps and plan sexual intimacy when you are well rested.

The incorporation of time and stress management skills is vital. We have become a nation of overworked, overscheduled, stressed individuals too busy for sexual intimacy. Sometimes it is important to schedule alone time to recharge your personal energy. Others find it helpful to schedule time for sex and intimacy. Sexual intimacy needs to become a priority for you and your partner. Set limits on other commitments such as employment, social responsibilities, and family obligations. Refocus your energies on your partner and your intimate time together. Sexual connectedness will help your overall health and improve your ability to handle many of life's challenges.

Similarly, you may be given specific sexually structured tasks to identify and help treat specific sexual complaints. Some examples of behavior modification sexual techniques include the following:

- Erotic reading: Try reading an erotic novel in a quiet relaxed place. This may rekindle some sexual thoughts or interests.
- Sensate focusing: Concentrate on your physical sensations. (This is discussed in further detail later.)
- Squeeze–stop techniques: This technique may be helpful for men with erectile concerns or premature ejaculation. The squeeze technique is when a man or his partner squeezes the **penis** before the point of ejaculatory inevitability. The stop–start technique is when the man stops stimulation as he senses getting closer to the point of ejaculatory inevitability.

Penis

The erectile, sexually, erotically sensitive organ in males. The penis serves a sexual function and also mediates the voiding of urine.

- Guided imagery: Imagine a particular sexual scenario.
- Relaxation techniques: Breathing and exercises may help you reconnect with your body and help lessen the stress you are experiencing.
- Exploration of sexual fantasies: Discussing sexual fantasies with your partner may help communication and eliminate sexual boredom. Some suggest using physical props like costumes or sexual accessories or mental imagery.
- Self-stimulation (**masturbation**) exercises: Self-stimulation is discussed later in Part Five.

You might be assigned homework in the form of sexual exploration. These activities may include nongenital touching, self-stimulation exercises, and other sexual exercises to improve and enhance your sexual self-esteem. You and your partner are educated through the use of open discussions concerning alternate forms of sexual expression, such as mutual massage, intimate fondling and caressing, and manual, digital, oral, and anal stimulation. Let your imagination be your guide.

Sometimes cueing exercises are also helpful. These exercises try to increase sexual self-esteem by helping you focus on a place and time in your life when you felt very sensual and sexy. Certain cues in the environment facilitate you looking and feeling attractive and sexy to others and yourself. Think back and try to remember your characteristics during this phase of your life. What was your hair like? Your body type or size? Your favorite scent or perfume? Music you enjoyed, or diet you enjoyed? It is likely that these cues are the key to your sense of sensuality and sexiness. Take a moment and write them down on a piece of paper. Think about incorporating them into your present-day routine and lifestyle. By association, you may feel that your sexual interest is rekindled.

You and your partner may be encouraged to engage in alternative sexual positions. Most couples engage in intercourse in the missionary position, which facilitates deep penetration. Some feel this is the best position in which to conceive a child

Masturbation

The act of self-pleasuring; also known as self-stimulation.

Pearls for Treating Sexual Complaints

69

because deep penetration places sperm near the cervix. But this position can sometimes be very painful for women who have shortened vaginas in association with vaginal and vulvar atrophy; rarely is the G-spot stimulated either.

Sexual intercourse in alternative positions may include side-to-side (spooning) or female-superior positions, where the woman is on top. These positions may help limit deep pelvic thrusting and minimize vaginal discomfort during penetration. Sometimes shallow thrusts or varying the depth, force, and vigor of movement can also change excitation and arousal. Some other sexual positions facilitate direct clitoral stimulation, which can greatly increase arousal in many women. If movement and mobility are issues, such as with chronic arthritis, bone and/or joint illness, osteoporosis, or fibromyalgia, use pillows or down comforters to help create a comfortable sexual situation. Use them liberally to support your body, back, and pelvis to avoid muscle strain.

41. What are some other sexual exercises?

Sexual exercises are often prescribed by the managing sexual healthcare professional or therapist and are used to reintroduce a couple to sexual exploration. Exercises may also enhance emotional connectedness and lead to a greater sense of emotional bonding.

Exercises may also enhance emotional connectedness and lead to a greater sense of emotional bonding.

According to the Sinclair Intimacy Institute, sensate focus exercises are a series of specific exercises for couples to perform that encourage each partner to take turns paying increased attention to their own senses. Sensate focus exercises can be used in therapy or at home and were originally developed by Masters and Johnson to help couples reconnect as they were experiencing sexual problems. These exercises, as well as the ones listed previously, can intensify personal sexual awareness and ultimately lead to increased connection and emotionality for couples.

A sensate focus exercise may be divided into several phases. Nonsexual stroking encourages both you and your partner to learn how to give and receive pleasure simply by touching each other's bodies; sexual penetration is discouraged and you should focus on caressing and pleasuring with a heightened sense of arousal and attentiveness. Increased awareness of sensations is paramount, and you both should take notice of body textures, temperatures, and contours while doing the touching. There is no pressure to perform need- or goal-oriented behavior such as orgasmic release, but you are encouraged to guide one another to sensual areas on your body and focus on pleasure and touch.

Sexual caresses and genital **foreplay** include touching and exploring the genital area (including breasts for women) of each other and guiding each other as to what is pleasurable and what sensations are less exciting. Open shared communication is encouraged and desired in these exercises. The man should educate his partner about the touch and pressure he enjoys on his penis, and you should also educate your partner about your sexual needs and give feedback on caresses and touch. Sexual penetration is not encouraged during this exercise, so if an **erection** occurs, it should be allowed to subside without orgasm and exercises should then be resumed. The Sinclair Institute discusses the ideas of the "hand riding" technique where you each place your hand on top of your partner's hand while being touched. This way you can indicate when you would like more or less pressure. You can also guide the rhythm to be faster or slower and even guide your lover to a different or erogenous or erotic body location.

Coital exercises are the next progressive step where you can engage in sexual penetration in a comfortable, nondemanding fashion and can continue to communicate and discuss sexual feelings and provide feedback to each other should issues or concerns arise. At some point, the female-on-top position is assumed and you can gently rub your partner's penis against your clitoral region, vulva, and vaginal opening. You may progress to putting his penis into your vagina if he has an erection, while focusing on the physical sensations. After completing

Foreplay

Sexual behavior engaged in during the early part of the sexual encounter, with the aim at intensifying sexual arousal or pleasure.

Erection

The expansion and hardening or stiffening of the sexual organ; it may be the penis, clitoris, or nipples in response to sexual fantasy or stimulation.

several attempts at this stage, couples are usually comfortable enough to proceed to intercourse.

Sensate focus exercises can be wonderful and liberating sensual and sexual experiences whereby you have given yourself permission to experience and give pleasure.

42. How do soft addictions such as compulsive use of iPods, Blackberries, cellular telephones, and computer laptops exert their effects on female sexuality and intimacy?

According to my blog at Revolutionhealth.com, cell phones and other advances in technology that have been invented to create free time in fact increase workloads and may affect sexual intimacy. It seems like everyone has a cell phone these days, and we often wonder what we did without such conveniences before they were invented. Cell phones, Blackberries, pagers, laptops, and other electronic equipment seem to keep us linked with the office and our work 24/7. But where does it end?

Many men and women have even developed soft additions or become compulsive checkers, unable to control their strong urges to be connected electronically and up to the minute with their e-mail. New medical syndromes are associated with finger and thumb problems as a result of increased typing and texting. Are you suffering from soft addictions to technological devices? The image of partners in bed clicking away on their respective Blackberries while the television drones in the background is not an uncommon bedroom scene. Some even are in the same home but e-mail each other from room to room. Clearly, we all need technology to help in our workday and to keep in touch with colleagues, but have we gone too far?

Are you suffering from soft addictions to technological devices?

All these technological activities help to an extent with time management, but the line between regular and compulsive use is a fine one. Many are overusing these devices and taking precious time away from their families and friends. Try to turn off every electronic device at a set time every night. (Although your inbox may be filled by morning, the truth is it will probably never be empty, no matter how hard you try.) Set limits on usage and stick to them. Don't cave. Share with your partner, communicate the old-fashioned way: have a discussion, face-to-face. Engage in intimacy in the moment and do not allow yourself to be interrupted. It takes work to overcome bad habits, and as with any addiction you may have a relapse, but if you want sexual intimacy to be a priority, you and your partner need to begin to try to kick the soft addiction habit! Soft addictions can limit intimacy and take away from time spent together as a couple. Limit use of convenience devices to a specific time frame and monitor your time spent on them so that it does not hinder sexual intimacy and inter-personal communication.

43. What is Tantra and how can it help sexual intimacy?

Tantra is the ancient Indian spiritual tradition and belief system that sexuality is tied to personal energy. Practicing Tantra, according to Tantric experts, can change us if we submit to our primal sexual desires while maintaining control and heightening spiritual awareness. When incorporated into lovemaking, Tantric techniques ultimately intensify the sexual dynamic or consciousness between partners as they fully experience their sensual and sexual energy together. Spiritual connections ensue and partners often relay experiences of sexual energy flowing from one partner to the next. Sexual enhancement, pleasuring, living consciously, and the various postures of lovemaking are important tenets of Tantra. The union of the male and female dimensions, or the yin and yang, expands the dimensions of sexuality. Through the control of orgasms, feelings of intimacy and connectedness with your partner are ultimately enhanced.

In Tantra, the ultimate sexual goal is to reach union on a spiritual plane and become one being. Sex therapy specialists

Tantra
An ancient Indian spiritual tradition and belief system with the premise that sexuality is tied into personal energy and is capable of changing us if we submit to our primal sexual desires while maintaining control and heightening spiritual awareness. Tantra can intensify lovemaking and intensify the sexual dynamic or consciousness between couples.

In Tantra, the ultimate sexual goal is to reach union on a spiritual plane and become one being.

who specialize in Tantra techniques are located in most areas of the United States. Dr. Lana Holstein and Dr. David Taylor offer an excellent sexual intimacy workshop at the Miraval Life in Balance Spa in Arizona. Through lectures and workshops, their program teaches couples to reconnect sexually, thus reclaiming sexual enrichments and satisfaction by exploring sexual pleasure and passion. Further information about their programs is on the Internet (www. miravalresort.com). According to Holstein and Taylor, there are techniques for couples that involve sitting silently face-to-face breathing together while the inner thought process is one of appreciation. Another important exercise is when the woman sits on her partner's lap with her legs wrapped around her partner's back to bring their hearts together, and the couple breathes together or alternately, almost as if each person is "breathing the other." These simple techniques are sensual, invigorating, and stimulating because they create profound intimacy and allow the formation of strong bonding connections between lovers.

Tantric practices can also be much more complicated, utilizing concepts of energy centers in the body, stressing the practices of nonejaculatory orgasms for men, and ejaculatory orgasms for women, as well as prolongation of intercourse with attention to building and ebbing of sexual energy. Tantra for the beginner should focus on intention to reach soulful, spiritual sexual exchange.

Dr. Laura Berman of the Berman Center (www.Theberman center.com) also offers intensive retreats for individuals and couples where the stress of everyday life is left behind and the focus becomes on jump-starting their sexual lives. Therapy, homework, and assigments focus on conflict resolution, increased communication, and other methods like tantra to enhance and reconnect sexually and spiritually.

44. What is mindfulness training?

Many of us travel on preprogrammed, unthinking autopilot, going to work, going through the motions without really paying attention to our surroundings or our own reactions. We are actually very often deep into a phase of life often called "mindlessness." We go home, check e-mail, cook dinner, and attend to the children all at the same time. Undoubtedly, we shoot off e-mail messages containing spelling errors or reply harshly without thought or consideration when we should have pondered our response. We cut our fingers chopping lettuce or miss the joyful smile of the coy, crafty toddler getting into mischief. We are on overload.

The habit of inattention, going through the motions or having your brain race with thoughts, leads us to not be ever present in our daily lives. We often ignore or dismiss important information and messages from our relationships, our friends, our own health, and even our own life. We can zone out, tune out, and shut the world down almost automatically when stress or conflict invades our lives.

Practicing the art of mindfulness is the key to being in the here-and-now, focusing on the present moment—using all of your focused senses in a challenged dynamic thought process. Sight, smell, touch, taste, and hearing all work in unison to create a whole image and picture of the process. Stop and smell the roses, but appreciate the hue of redness, the texture of the leaves, the imperfections of the petals, and the sparkling fragrance of the unique flower.

Dr. Lori Brotto, noted sexual health researcher, and some of her Vancouver colleagues have published extensively on the notion of mindfulness and its use in the treatment of female sexual dysfunction disorders. The concept of focusing on bodily functions and performance can help women a great deal in understanding their body's normative function. Intense focusing on self can also help to solidify and enhance sexual

The habit of inattention, going through the motions or having your brain race with thoughts, leads us to not be ever present in our daily lives.

Pearls for Treating Sexual Complaints

constructs and thoughts. Brotto and her esteemed colleagues have shown this technique of mindfulness training to be effective in patients with malignancies and sexual complaints. Mindfulness training has also been helpful in treating a variety of other medical conditions and may be helpful in chronic pain syndromes.

Try some relaxation techniques such as deep breathing and resting comfortably in silence with serene quietness. Pay attention without letting your mind wander or trying to change any thought. Be aware. Stop and smell and touch and feel and appreciate the rose petals in their universe and specific environmental context. Stay in the present, and if you wander, let yourself drift back to your original thought. Focus on your deep breathing, each breath as it enters and exits your lungs, before an activity, and think about the experience. You can expect your mind to wander or deviate from the concentration course with intrusive or conflicting thoughts, but slowly, thoughtfully, and gently bring it back to the concentrated ideal or experience.

Try to anchor your awareness in the present moment. Stay focused and try not to let your mind wonder. Stay focused on the present moment, not on the future or the "what-ifs" or "whats" that life may bring. Begin by trying to narrow your focus of thought and begin to appreciate your individual thoughts and ideals. Your mind will become clearer and senses more heightened. You will be in the moment during sexual intimacy and feel a deeper sense of connection both to your inner sexual self and your partner's sensuality.

Do not expect to achieve a state of mindfulness overnight—it is a process of practice and dedication. The more you focus your mind and channel your energies, the easier it will become for future endeavors.

Yoga, meditation, and even acupuncture may be helpful in the treatment of sexual complaints. New data are emerging about these stress and relaxation techniques, and many find help by incorporating them into their treatment plan.

45. What is sexual education or bibliotherapy, and how can it help with my sexual function?

Women often are not aware of sexual responsiveness and genital anatomy. Understanding your genital anatomy, what it looks and feels like, will help you know your normal physiologic response and how sexual arousal occurs. As a first step, examine your genitals with the aid of a handheld mirror alone or in the presence of a sexual healthcare professional. Do you know where the clitoral tissue is located? Touch the vagina lips, feel the contour of the vaginal walls. Can you properly identify all the parts of your anatomy? This is the beginning of your sexual education. Focusing on other literature or **erotica** may also be helpful in broadening your sexual experience and understanding.

Have you ever wondered where they keep the "magazines for women"? Where are the pictures of naked men? Next time you travel, look at the local newsstand; you're sure to find numerous magazines marketed to men—you can possibly decipher many familiar titles under the protective plastic or boards covering the erotically charged pictures. Published data support the premise that erotica and sexually explicit movies and pictures and pornography visually stimulate men more than women. Women, on the other hand, are less visually stimulated. Some women do tell of increased sexual interest and desire for sexual intimacy after reading erotically charged literature, but almost uniformly women are not as stimulated by sexually visual material as men are.

One of the exercises that your sexual healthcare professional may prescribe is *bibliotherapy*. Bibliotherapy consists of many take-home items, such as pamphlets, books, videos, and other visual aids, that provide educational instruction or reinforcement for you and your partner. These materials may also serve

Erotica
Sexually themed work such as books or sculpture deemed to have literary and artistic merit. Naked men, women, and other body parts are often featured as predominant themes.

Have you ever wondered where they keep the "magazines for women"?

as a future guide or reference. Many are graphic and have a variety of pictures demonstrating sexual positioning while others are narratives.

The Internet has become a main educational resource for women who suffer from sexual complaints. Women are thirsty for accurate, easily readable information. The Women's Sexual Health Foundation (www.twshf.org), founded by Lisa Martinez, is an excellent resource for patients and serves as an advocacy group for women's sexual health care. The International Society for the Study of Women's Sexual Health (ISSWSH), the premier organization for women's sexual health at www.isswsh.org; the North American Menopause Society (NAMS, www.menopause.org); and the American College of Obstetricians and Gynecologists (ACOG, www.acog.org) are all organizations that maintain current information on their websites concerning sexual health and sexual education. They also provide medical information about the latest updates on female sexual therapeutics. For the female cancer survivor, the American Cancer Society's booklet titled *Cancer and Sexuality* is an excellent patient reference guide. It provides factual information and helpful suggestions to maintain and improve your sexual functioning.

Be certain to contact a reputable organization when you are seeking information and sexual education. Make sure the data are up-to-date and that the authors are reputable healthcare providers in the field of sexual medicine.

46. What is an erotic reading list?

Dr. Susan Kellogg-Spadt, codirector of the Pelvic and Sexual Health Institute Sexual Medicine Institute in Philadelphia, has developed an exciting and enticing erotic reading list. This is a listing of some important erotically charged, sexually explicit material that can be helpful in the comprehensive treatment of female sexual complaints. Sexual research has verified that women who read erotic literature, either instructional or fantasy, have more spontaneous sexual thoughts and fantasies. They may also be experiencing more satisfying sexual behavior than are women who do not.

Enjoying erotic literature is a perfectly normal part of nourishing your sexual soul. Your interest in certain sexual fantasy does not necessarily represent your desire for certain activities in your real life. Many sexual medicine professionals may request that you purchase a few of the books on an erotic reading list and commit to reading them at least 15 to 20 minutes three times per week. When you are reading, you should be alone, relaxed, and in a private place without distractions. Table 1 lists a few of Dr. Kellogg-Spadt's suggestions.

Table 1 Instructional and Fantasy Reading materials

Instructional Reading	Fantasy Reading
Becoming Orgasmic (Heiman & LaPicolo)	*The Best New Erotica* (Caroll & Groff)
The Elusive Orgasm (Cass)	*Aqua Erotica* (Mohanraj)
The Busy Couple's Guide to Great Sex (McAllister & Rallie)	*The Blue Moon Erotic Reader* (Burner & Russet)
The Art of Kissing (Cane)	*Erotic Interludes* (Barbach)
The Big O (Paget)	*Forbidden Flowers My Secret Garden* (Friday)
Sex for One/Orgasm for Two (Dodson)	*Erotic Edge/Pleasures* (Barbach)
The G Spot (Whipple et al.)	*Historical Erotica* (Carroll & Groff)
Resurrecting Sex (Schnarch)	*Herotica* (Bright)
The Good Girl's Guide to Bad Girl Sex (Keesling)	*Erotic Fairy Tales* (Szereto)
Satisfaction: Women, Sex, and the Quest for Intimacy (Clayton & Robin)	
Getting the Sex You Want (Leiblum)	

Another title to add to an erotic reading list is *The Ultimate Guide to Adult Videos: How to Watch Adult Videos and Make Your Sex Life Sizzle*. In this book, Violet Blue, sex educator, reviews countless DVDs, and it is perfect for the adult-video neophyte.

Some other suggestions include *Real Sex for Real Women* by Dr. Laura Berman, an excellent book with color picture that helps every woman, no matter what shape or size combine the realities of everyday life with satisfying sexual passion. Dr. Berman also has an extensive list of home DVDs that can help spice up your sexual life.

Celebrating Orgasm: Women's Private Self-Loving Sessions, is an excellent DVD by famous sexologist Betty Dodson. The DVD guides five women (ages 26 to 62) through overcoming their concerns, fears, and inhibitions about self-stimulation techniques. It offers suggestions for a variety of clitoral stimulation methods and is an excellent teaching tool to help women experience orgasmic arousal. *The Passion and Power: The Technology of Orgasm* is a documentary produced and directed by Wendy Slick and Emiko Omori. It explores the dynamic connection between the vibrator and the female orgasm.

47. How do I know if I need psychosexual therapy and counseling?

Because women's sexual complaints are complex phenomena and situational issues are a fundamental part of the diagnosis, a comprehensive treatment regime includes appropriate sexual counseling and therapy. A certified sexual therapist who is educated and trained to deal with patients with sexual complaints is often the best mental healthcare provider to treat sexual complaints. These specialists are qualified to deal with psychosexual issues that include body image, changes in intimacy, sexuality, self-esteem, and mood.

You may also need marital, individual, couples, and/or group therapy, depending on your need and specific complaint. In general, most patients can benefit from brief psychosexual interventions that include education, counseling/support, and symptom management. Psychotherapists and psychologists can be extremely effective when **vaginal dilators** are prescribed for the treatment of vaginismus and other painful sexual syndromes where a woman's vaginal muscles close tightly almost involuntarily.

Seeking treatment of both the medical and psychological concerns of a sexual complaint with close collaboration between the medical clinician and psychosexual therapist can help alleviate your sexual symptoms. You may be required to sign release forms so that your sexual medicine specialist can discuss your case with the therapist, and vice versa. Frequent visits to your sexual healthcare team are often needed to help with sexual complaints and pain syndromes like dyspareunia, vulvodynia, and vaginismus.

Local and national support organizations such as the American Association for Sex Education, Counseling and Treatment (AASECT, www.aasect.org) and Association of Reproductive Health Professionals (ARHP) can provide further information and support to help you achieve greater comfort with these issues, within your relationships and families and within yourself.

Vaginal dilators
Medical applications that can be placed within the vagina to help restore the vaginal tissues so that they are more adaptable.

Seeking treatment of both the medical and psychological concerns of a sexual complaint with close collaboration between the medical clinician and psychosexual therapist can help alleviate your sexual symptoms.

Pearls for Treating Sexual Complaints

PART FIVE

Sex for One: The Art of Self-Stimulation

What are some important facts about self-pleasure and stimulation?

What is a vibrator or self-stimulator?

What is the G-spot? Does it really exist?

More . . .

48. What is the history of masturbation?

Autogratification (self-stimulation or masturbation) was condemned as an evil taboo in many cultures and throughout many historical eras. It was seen as a cause of medical illness and viewed as an activity that weakened the soul and the mind. However, during the ancient period of Greek hedonism, sexual enjoyment and expression were encouraged and advocated. Masturbation was regarded as a natural activity if men could not find other copulation opportunities. This philosophy was in contradiction to the emerging 18th-century preoccupation with self-pleasure and anti-masturbatory doctrine. Victorian intellects quoted the Bible and asserted that masturbation was self-abuse. The medicalization of the Judeo-Christian view of masturbation, viewing it as an illness, became prevalent in the 18th century. Physicians became moral leaders and attempted to tackle controversial issues masturbation.

The concept of masturbation as an illness was first described in an anonymous 18th-century English document in Holland, *"Onania": The Heinous Sin of Self-Pollution*. Spilling semen through masturbation was viewed as the cause of a wide range of medical and psychological illnesses: skin ailments like pustules and acne; digestive diseases including nausea, vomiting, constipation; deteriorating eyesight, hearing, and sense of smell; and various nervous conditions. James Graham (1745–1794), a self-proclaimed sex therapist, also depicted masturbation as the primary cause destroying the mind and body. Masturbation was unnatural, and autoerotica became synonymous with medical pathology, madness, mania, dementia, and melancholy and could lead to suicide. Masturbators were thought to have frail offspring. Children were often victims of the masturbation policy; their self-exploration and discovery of their genitals were hindered, often with force and sophisticated gadgetry, to prevent auto-stimulation.

In 1860, articles in American medical journals discussed a therapy to cure masturbation invented by a prominent British physician, Isaac Brown-Baker, who pioneered the operative procedure of clitorectomy (removal of the clitoris) for female neuroses, hysteria, and epilepsy. Although many American and European medical professionals condemned this procedure, it was still utilized in many instances in a gallant attempt to treat many for their bizarre ailments. Others advocated the blistering of the vulva and thighs and the lyses of clitoral adhesions or **female circumcision** to prevent female masturbation. Male masturbators were not exempt from therapy; they were locked in straightjackets, genital cages, and penile rings with sharp points on the inside to inhibit nocturnal emissions.

It was not until Kinsey's revolutionary 1948 study that the philosophy of masturbation changed. This study of sexual behavior revealed that close to 92% of men and close to 58% of women masturbate to orgasm as some point in their lives. Masturbation was reborn; it was systematically disconnected from perversion, insanity, impotence, and medical or psychological illness. Many still believe that masturbation is a necessary step in developing into a normal, sexual, orgasmic being. Masturbation was even regarded as an acceptable activity in a marital relationship; it was seen as individual exploration of one's own sexuality and a highly personal outlet.

Although society has progressed in many ways, the philosophy and social taboos associated with masturbation are still prevalent. For instance, in 1970 Mark Peterson of the Council of the Twelve Apostles wrote *The Mormon Guide to Overcoming Masturbation*, a 21-point manifesto to help Mormons keep their hands out of their pants. The position today of the Roman Catholic Church remains that masturbation is an intrinsically and gravely disordered action. The sexual guilt and fear associated with being found out as a masturbator can in fact cause psychological and emotional damage, the Church believes.

Female circumcision

Any form of ritualized genital cutting or excision or destruction of parts of the female genitalia.

Although society has progressed in many ways, the philosophy and social taboos associated with masturbation are still prevalent.

Sex for One: The Art of Self-Stimulation

In our present day, in the face of sexually transmitted diseases, masturbation can be advocated as the safest form of sexual activity besides celibacy. Masturbation has become an essential outlet for sexual tension and frustration and can help curb risk-taking behavior. Masturbation is often a man's first sexual activity and his most frequent activity; it can relieve psychological stress. Masturbation is sanctioned as an individualistic experience that can fulfill many varied needs for different people (the young, the old, and the timid may have no other sexual outlet). A pro-sex group in San Francisco has even declared that May be known as National Masturbation Month; May 7 was designated as Masturbation Day.

In one generation, masturbation moved from an abnormal behavior that results in madness and medical illness to a healthy activity that can promote sexual well-being and normal development. Prior to Kinsey, masturbation was a sin that made hair grow on the palms of boys and on the faces of girls. By dispelling the myths about masturbation, it can be promoted as an erotic activity that can promote a positive sexual self-image. The ecstasy of solo sex is ubiquitous and will continue to enhance human beings' sexual, erotic, and sensual repertoire.

Autoerotic
Providing sexual stimulation to oneself or being aroused sexually by oneself.

Bodily exploration and enjoyment of personal autoerotic behavior may be an important step in your sexual health and wellness.

49. What are some important facts about self-pleasure and stimulation?

Masturbation is the self-stimulation of your genitalia for sexual arousal and pleasure. Many unfavorable views concerning masturbation in our present-day society have a deep foundation in early history. Your healthcare provider may encourage sexual stimulation to arousal or orgasm so that you redevelop or experience pleasurable experiences associated with self-touch and intimacy. Bodily exploration and enjoyment of personal **autoerotic** behavior may be an important step in your sexual health and wellness.

Research has shown that self-stimulation is the most common sexual act:

- According to Leung in an article published in *Clinical Pediatrics*, 90–94% of men and 50–60% of women have self-stimulated at some point in time during their childhood or adolescence. Many continue well into adulthood and old age.
- Women enjoy self-pleasure and autoeroticism, maybe not as often as men do, but it does exist.
- Masturbation is not associated with any medical illnesses or psychological defects or disease.
- Many people in healthy, committed relationships continue to masturbate and continue to explore their bodies and enjoy areas of self-pleasure.
- Accidental autoerotic asphyxia (attempts to limit oxygen intake whereby self-inflicting noose-like apparatuses are created to enhance sexual pleasure) deaths are on the rise.

50. What is the Eros Clitoral Stimulator?

The Eros Clitoral Stimulator is a sexual device produced by Urometrics that is FDA approved for the treatment of female sexual dysfunction. It is available by prescription only and has been used for patients who have had cervical cancer and other pelvic cancers, such as rectal and vaginal cancers. This devise has been studied in a small population of cervical cancer patients. It is a handheld device that has a small suction cup at its tip. This tip seals around the clitoral area, creates a vacuum, and facilitates blood draw and vasocongestion in the clitoral region. The device has been shown to be helpful with clitoral engorgement and may be helpful with orgasmic and arousal disorders or complaints. Preliminary medical data show promising results that this device might be helpful in combating arousal difficulties after radiation in the pelvis, especially in cervical cancer patients. In other populations, such as women who have diabetes or other neuropathies, this device may also be helpful. Ask your healthcare provider if this device is right for you.

The device is, however, costly and is available only by prescription. Insurance plans vary and many will pay for it; however, others will not. Check with your insurance carrier to see if your policy will cover the expense. If you think this device will help you and be useful in your treatment for sexual dysfunction, ask your sexual healthcare provider for more information.

51. What is a vaginal dilator and how do I use one?

Women who have undergone pelvic surgery or who suffer from vaginal shortening, vaginal narrowing, or scar tissue that may interfere or prevent penetration (and cause vaginal pain) have pelvic discomfort that makes them avoid sexual behavior. Vaginal dilators, or inserts, may be prescribed as part of their sexual rehabilitation regime. These dilators are size-graded vaginal inserts usually made of plastic or silicone; they are inserted into the vaginal canal. Dilators are often used to facilitate lengthening and widening of the vagina. They may also be used to help stretch the vaginal scar tissue that may contribute to pain and discomfort of vaginal intercourse.

Dilators can be used on a regular basis and with water- or hormone-based lubricants. The suggested schedules range from once daily for 10 to 15 minutes to at least three times weekly. Several studies report that ongoing supportive behavioral therapy is instrumental for continued compliance. Just getting a dilator is not enough—you need to see your sexual healthcare provider on a regular basis to ensure that you make slow but steady progress. Start off using the smallest size and gradually work up to the next larger size once you are comfortable.

To use a vaginal dilator, first begin by preparing yourself and your environment for dilator therapy. Make certain you will have privacy either by locking your door or working with your dilator when you will not be interrupted. At the Southern California Center for Sexual Health and Survivorship Medicine, we advocate using the dilators in the morning hours just before starting the day. This suggestion is for several reasons. Trying to do this at night often doesn't work for the active, vibrant woman. At the end of a long, busy day with work, family, and social obligations, many women believe that it is too time consuming to do the dilator therapy. Too often fatigue and rest supersede sexual rehabilitation. Another reason to do dilator therapy in the morning is that after completion, you can shower and clean off and prepare for your day. Showering after therapy can be helpful if the lubricant is messy and/or results in any vaginal leakage. It only takes a few extra minutes.

The dilator should be inserted into the vagina with a generous amount of water-based lubricant. You should lie on your back, bend your knees, and spread your knees apart. With gentle pressure, the vaginal dilator should be inserted into the vagina as deeply as possible while still maintaining some comfort. Try to leave the dilator in place for about 10 to 15 minutes while remaining on your back. It is often helpful to be distracted by other activities while the dilator is in place, such as reading a book or watching television. After removing the dilator, it is important to wash it with warm water and soap, dry it with clean towel, and store it in a safe secure place.

Stay at one size for a least one week and ensure that there is no pain or discomfort, and then try the next size. Remember that it is a process and stepwise—Rome was not build in a day! Often it takes time to advance. If you feel that your muscles are tensing up, practice some self-talking exercises and focus on your conscious awareness that you are in control of the dilator and muscle relaxation. Try to relax tense muscles—take deep breaths in and out and focus on relaxation. Ease up on your pressure on the dilator and make certain that you have used enough lubricant.

Dilators can be very helpful in a variety of clinical situations. Be certain to discuss them and your progress with your sexual healthcare provider.

52. What is a vibrator or self-stimulator?

You can purchase many sexual accessories to help stimulate your erogenous zones and genitals. Some devices enhance pleasure while others are part of complex sexual medicine treatment plans. Women do enjoy vibratory sensations on their breasts, vulva, and clitoral tissues, and in the perianal area as well as the vaginal vault.

Steam-powered vibrating devices were patented in the 1860s and 1870s by George Taylor, and the first electromechanical vibrator was designed in 1880 by British physician Joseph Mortimer Granville (he intended it to be used for massage of male skeletal muscles). Doctors originally used vibrators, or self-stimulators, as a cure-all for female ailments: female hysteria, pelvic pain, nervous tension, and a wide variety of gynecologic complaints. In the 1920s, vibrators became associated with pornography and illicit sexuality, and only recently have sexual accessories and vibrators come to be viewed favorably as adjunctive medical accessories to help restore or enhance sexual response.

Vibrators come in a variety of shapes, sizes, and colors. Some have electrical cords, and others are battery operated. The intensity of stimulation varies between vibrators, and most have variable speeds and settings. These sexual devices can be helpful for women who may need extra vibratory stimulation on the sensitive erotic areas of the vagina, vulva, and clitoris. Vibrators have proven useful during self-stimulatory behavior and can also be used with your partner during sexual foreplay. Some are available for purchase over the Internet and at local sexual paraphernalia shops. Some sexual healthcare professionals even offer a variety of products that can be purchased in the privacy of the doctor's office. Self-stimulators, or **dildos**, can be used with water-based lubricants. It is important to

Dildo

A sexual toy that is often phallic in nature or shaped like a penis and that can be used to penetrate the vagina or anus. Both men and women often incorporate dildos into sexual play. Another term often used is vaginal/anal dilator.

keep them clean by washing them with warm water and soap using a sponge or cloth and rinsing well; cleaning after each use is always recommended, and the sharing of toys should be discouraged. Storage should be in a clean, private place, and most recommend removal of batteries during storage periods. It is important to note that silicone lubricant should not be used with silicone sexual accessories.

Vibrators can be used alone as part of self-erotic exploration and sexual play or as part of your sexual repertoire with your partner. Generally, sexual massagers can be used both internally and externally to enhance stimulation, arousal, and pleasure. You can stimulate the labia, vaginal tissue, and clitoral tissue and even enhance testicular or penile stimulation for your partner. If you share your sexual toys, then it is doubly important to cleanse them in between uses.

Vibrators can be used alone as part of self-erotic exploration and sexual play or as part of your sexual repertoire with your partner.

A variety of devices are extremely popular among women and have been reported to enhance sexual stimulation and orgasmic intensity. One new self-stimulator, the Adonis, created by the sexual expert and therapist Dr. Laura Berman, has gained popularity because it actively stimulates, simultaneously, both the clitoral region and the vaginal G-spot. The electronic stimulation device called Slight Touch is a battery-powered, over-the-counter device that uses electrodes applied to the top of the foot above the ankles and above the buttocks to stimulate nerve pathways to the genital areas. The Vivelle device is a battery-operated external clitoral stimulation device that is worn on the fingers and may help orgasm when used with a special lubricant. Some other very popular female sexual devices include The Rabbit, and The Pocket Rocket. Both are extremely popular among women and have been reported to enhance sexual stimulation and orgasmic intensity.

The Hitachi Magic Wand is also another popular and favorite for many women. It is also known as the Rolls Royce of vibrators and has a spongy-headed massager. The Rabbit is the bunny-earred vibrator that gained popularity from the

Sex for One: The Art of Self-Stimulation

women of the television series *Sex & the City*. Some of these vibrators have swirling shafts that can stimulate the sensitive vaginal opening and external rabbit ears that excite the clitoral tissues. The Pocket Rocket is approximately four-inches long and has been considered a mini-massager. It is quiet, discreet, and small but packs a lot of power. Many prefer this device since it can be easily transported during vacation time. Some others prefer it since partners can use this low-tech device without feeling threatened. I Rub My Ducky is a waterproof toy basically identical to the classic rubber ducky who once splashed around your bathtub. When you press down, a soothing one-speed vibrator begins. Rock Chick is similar to the Adonis described above as it is a U-shaped vibrator designed to arouse the G-spot and clitoris simultaneously.

You can often buy vibrators and other sexual accessories in stores that sell small appliances; they are often labeled as massagers. In addition to visiting your local sex store, which for some may be embarrassing or concerning, you can buy a vibrator in the comfort of your home on the Internet. Take the time to browse, read reviews, and check out pricing. Always ensure that the site you are purchasing from has a privacy agreement and make sure you won't be getting unwanted spam from it as well. Most will not put your name on mailing lists and will ensure discreet packaging when delivering the purchase to your home. Some of the more popular websites include www.drugstore.com, which offers home delivery of sexual accessories in a discreet manor and does not send unwanted e-mail or mailings; www.goodvibes.com; www.xandriacollections.com; and www.evesgarden.com.

53. What is the OhMiBod?

The latest craze in iPod technology has infiltrated the female sexual forum: the new electronic gadget called the OhMiBod is a vibrator that offers a whole new twist on how to enjoy your iPod. According to the website, "Everyone enjoys their own type of music and their unique musical beat. The OhMiBod combines music and pleasure to create the ultimate sexual experience." This sexual accessory is simple and easy to use—simply attach it to your existing iPod and enjoy the sensation of vibrations along with your musical tunes. It is heralded as more than just a pleasure toy because it "harnesses the iPod musical movement and popularity to bring a higher level of acceptance and openness about sexuality in a fun and liberating way. Young or old, single or partnered, people from all walks of life are experiencing an amazing new way to connect and share the pleasures of orgasmic play."

It is easy to order and arrives in a discrete package. Special accessories such as personal lubricant, garters, and other sexual enhancers can be purchased with the OhMiBod vibrator. The instructions are easy: simply plug the new OhMiBod into your existing iPod or any music player, and it automatically vibrates to the rhythm and intensity of the music. Relax and enjoy; let your body feels the vibrations as you get down with your favorite tunes. OhMiBod aficionados write about their experiences, trade tips, share their favorite play lists, and more. There is even a blog for OhMiBod users.

54. How do I use a self-stimulator?

Many different kinds of vibrators can be used for massage or sexual pleasure. They come in a variety of different sizes, shapes, and materials and can even be remote-control, clitoral, G-spot, or waterproof. They can be battery-powered or use an electrical outlet. For some women, a vibrator might make the difference between adequate stimulation and the ability to achieve an orgasm or not. About 60% of the female population are not able to reach an orgasm with penetration alone. If you have never used a vibrator, it may seem like a scary thing. Here are some helpful instructions for the novice or the expert alike.

Get to know your vibrator. Take your vibrator out of the package and get to know how it works and what kind of batteries it takes. Play with the buttons, turn it on and off, and examine switches. Find out how many speeds and settings it has. Wash your vibrator well before using it; use warm water with a mild soap and make sure to rinse it well so that no residual soap remains. If it isn't waterproof, be careful not to get any water near the battery case. Check for sharp edges or seams.

Start on your own. Even if you're planning on using your vibrator with a partner, it's a good idea to check it out by yourself first. You'll feel less self-conscious and you can really concentrate on how it feels. Make sure you have enough time and privacy. If you have roommates, children, thin walls, or nosy neighbors, you can always turn on some music, shut the blinds, and make use of blankets and comforters to mute the sound.

Play with the lights turned on. Not everyone will be comfortable with this suggestion. Playing with a vibrator with the lights on can be very educational and useful. You can discover specific places on your body that are rich with nerve endings and ready for enjoyment and stimulation. This is the kind of information you can use on yourself and in the future to share with a lover.

Turn it off before you turn it on. Get comfortable with the feel of the vibrator on your body. Run it along your body without even turning it on. Notice how it feels. Press it firmly against your skin and press it onto your body and massage your muscles. If the vibrator is made out of a hard material this will probably feel nice. If the vibrator is a soft rubber and doesn't feel smooth against your skin, try it with your clothes on. This isn't meant to give you an orgasm, but it's a gentle and nonthreatening way of introducing your body to the vibrator.

Move your vibrator from the outside in. Once you turn it on, start by touching the vibrator to your body to help you understand the vibration sensation. Even though vibrators are used mostly around the vulva and clitoris, get a feel for the vibration all over your body include touching your breasts and other areas where it will feel good. Slowly move to the more sensitive parts of your body.

Do not be in a rush: explore every part of your body. The interesting thing about vibrators is that they never get tired, and they let you explore every inch of your body for sexual pleasure. Many women use vibrators for clitoral stimulation, and some report that one side or even one portion of their clitoris responds to vibration more than another. Don't rush; leaving a vibrator in place can allow it to establish sensation connections that previously weren't there.

Adjust the speed, pressure, and other settings of the vibrator. Most vibrators have multiple speed settings (or at least two settings). Always start on a low setting and work your way up. Experiment with applying different pressures. You may enjoy a lot of deep pressure with clitoral stimulation.

Most women use vibrators for external stimulation, but as long as your vibrator is safe for penetration, there's no reason not to try it. A vibrator that is safe for penetration will be smooth, have no rough edges, and won't absorb bodily fluids. In almost all cases, it's recommended to put a condom over a vibrator if you're using it for penetration. You should also use water-based lubricant when using a vibrator for penetration. If you are not sharing your vibrator and are using it exclusively for yourself, then you may choose not use a condom.

Start slow with penetration and get yourself aroused by using the vibrator externally first. Although far more nerve endings are outside the vagina than inside, lots of women enjoy penetration with a vibrator. Some women will use a vibrator to stimulate the G-spot (see Question 55). It has also been hypothesized that nerve endings in the cervix respond to stimulation and pressure. Pressing the vibrator against the top of your vagina (such as pressing it toward your belly) may provide G-spot stimulation or even indirect clitoral stimulation.

You can use your vibrator with your partner in any number of ways. You can control the pressure, using it on yourself to add stimulation during sex play with a partner. You can use the vibrator on your partner (or vice versa). You can also find

You can use your vibrator with your partner in any number of ways.

Sex for One: The Art of Self-Stimulation

a vibrator that fits well between you and your partner that neither of you need to control, but that can add stimulation during sex. If you want to insert a vibrator for penetration be certain that the toy is smooth and seamless. Also be certain to use a condom if you are using the vibrator with another partner or sharing the toy.

Take your batteries out. Get in the habit of taking your batteries out of the vibrator each time you are finished using it. If you leave the batteries in, the vibrator may turn on to a very low speed (or you may leave it on low without knowing it) and this can both burn out the motor and make for some embarrassing moments when everyone at dinner is wondering where that buzzing sound is coming from. Also, if you leave your vibrator alone for extended periods with the batteries in, they can corrode and leak into the battery case, destroying your vibrator.

55. What is the G-spot? Does it really exist?

Gräfenberg spot (G-spot)

An area of increased erotic sensitivity on or deep in the front of the vagina. It is located on the anterior surface of the vaginal vault. Stimulation in some women provides intense sexual pleasure.

The **Gräfenberg spot**, more familiarly known and referred to as the G-spot, is named after the Berlin-based gynecologist Ernst Gräfenberg, who first published an article in the *International Journal of Sexology* in 1950 titled "The Role of Urethra in Female Orgasm." In this article, Gräfenberg proposes that the clitoris is not the sole anatomic structure responsible for female sexual arousal, lending a concrete anatomic structure to the theories of vaginal orgasm. In his gynecologic examination of women, Gräfenberg reported the discovery that "an erotic zone . . . could be demonstrated on the anterior wall of the vagina along the course of the urethra." The G-spot was subsequently popularized by Ladas, Whipple, and Perry with the publication of their ground-breaking book on female sexuality, *The G-Spot and Other Recent Discoveries About Human Sexuality*, and it has become known as an erogenous zone that, when stimulated, leads to high levels of sexual arousal and powerful orgasms.

Because the initial evidence for the existence of the G-spot was based almost exclusively on anecdotal evidence, several scientific investigators in the mid- to late 1980s sought to more rigorously and methodically evaluate the subject matter. Hoch and associates studied vaginal erotic sensitivity in 56 women by a sexologic examination of the vagina tissues. The female subjects in this study were selected from a group of 59 couples who were experiencing sexual complaints related to **anorgasmia,** or the inability to achieve orgasm. Sexologic examination included a detailed gynecologic and physical examination involving digital exploration of the vaginal walls by a trained healthcare provider while the patient was asked to take note of the variations in sensation throughout different locations within the vagina. Rather than finding one single erogenous spot, Hoch and associates concluded that the entire anterior vaginal wall was erotically sensitive in most female subjects.

Many researchers believe that the G-spot is not a specific discrete structure, but rather a collection of erogenous zones primarily located on the upper anterior wall as well as in the lower posterior vaginal wall. This is an area inside the vagina that is extremely sensitive to deep pressure. Davidson and colleagues anonymously questioned 2350 professional women about their personal perception of their own sexual anatomy. Of the 1245 women who responded, 84.3% believed that an exceptionally powerful and sensitive area existed within the vagina. The perceived areas of location were varied among the respondents, however, including anterior vaginal wall (55.1%), posterior vaginal wall (7.3%), upper vagina (46.1%), and lower vagina (21.5%).

Female Ejaculation

Many sexual healthcare providers believe that when properly stimulated, the G-spot can swell and lead to orgasm in many women. At the time of orgasm, many ejaculate through the urethra some liquid that is chemically similar to male ejaculate but that contains no sperm.

Anorgasmia

Difficulty experiencing or the inability to experience orgasm; in women it is often referred to as female orgasmic disorder.

Sex for One: The Art of Self-Stimulation

Approximately 10–40% of women ejaculate, and the quantity may be from a sprinkle to a gush, drops to tablespoons; most women may exude rather than spurt fluid. The fluid or ejaculate is from the urethra and occurs during orgasm. It is often ignored by obstetricians and gynecologists, and many women confuse this with urination. The link between the G-spot and **female ejaculation** originates from Gräfenberg's original paper that noted the possible existence of such a phenomenon in response to female sexual arousal and orgasm. Chemical analysis of female ejaculate was shown to have higher levels of prostatic acid phosphatase than preorgasmic urine samples as well as significantly lower urea and creatinine levels.

Female ejaculation

Expulsion from the urethra in women of about 3 to 5 milliliters of fluid different in chemical composition from urine.

56. What is G-spot enhancement or amplification?

G-spot amplification (GSA) is a novel method of augmenting the G-spot using cosmetic tissue filler such as human-engineered collagen or hyaluronic acid (Restylane). The premise of these interventions is that the injection enlarges the G-spot, making it easier to locate and henceforth stimulate. The cosmetic procedure has been touted as a method for enhancing female arousal and female subjective experience of orgasm. Centers offering this procedure claim that one intervention may last approximately 3 to 6 months. It is not covered by insurance and is extremely costly. Patients must also sign extensive consent forms.

As of yet, there have been no randomized, controlled studies on efficacy, safety, or side effect profile for this cosmetic procedure. There exists much controversy as to whether or not cosmetic procedures should be done based upon patient autonomy to improve and/or enhance sexual function. Caution should be exercised before considering this procedure. It is best to seek out a professional sexual medicine specialist for a comprehensive history and physical examination prior to considering this operation.

PART SIX

Sexual Pharmacology

What is vaginal dryness and how does it affect
sexuality? What can be done?

What are estrogen creams?

What is testosterone replacement and how is it linked
with women's sexuality?

More . . .

Hormones are often considered mainstay interventions that can improve sexual function. Systemic and local hormonal replacement with estrogen, progesterone, and testosterone remain key components in the management of female sexual dysfunction. Estrogen is one of many important hormones that is necessary for sexual function in women. Central arousal in the brain, peripheral tissues, and pelvic sexual region is dependent on estrogen levels. Some tissues are also very dependent on testosterone levels. Systemic hormonal replacement can be achieved with a variety of products either taken orally (by mouth), transdermally (through a skin patch), or intravaginally (in the vagina). There are many products on the market and they come in a variety of strengths and with different delivery systems—there are pills, gels, rings, tablets, and mists, among others. It is always critical to discuss your specific health background with your medical provider to decide what is best for you. Some of the popular hormones are Premarin, PremPro (Wyeth Pharmaceuticals), Activella (Novonordisk), and Vivelle Dot (Novartis). Creams include Premarin Vaginal Cream (Wyeth Pharmaceuticals) and Estrace Cream (Warner Chicott Pharmaceuticals).

Progestin

A synthetic form of progesterone often used in birth control pills and hormone therapy.

For women who have an intact uterus, the standard of medical care is to add a **progestin** agent to the regime; this prevents endometrial hyperplasia, or overgrowth of the uterine lining, and is widely accepted to help in the prevention of endometrial cancer. With the emerging data from the Woman's Health Initiative study, whereby hormones have had a small linkage to the possible development of cancer, there are growing concerns about hormones and potential associated risks of cardiovascular events or breast cancer. Risks and benefit profiles should be discussed with your healthcare and sexual medicine specialist.

Vaginal atrophy/ dryness is a serious medical issue associated with a drop in estrogen levels in the genital area.

57. What is vaginal dryness and how does it affect sexuality? What can be done?

Vaginal atrophy/ dryness is a serious medical issue associated with a drop in estrogen levels in the genital area. Many women suffer in silence with this condition. It can lead to decreased vaginal elasticity, pliability, and stretchability. Many women with severe atrophy or dryness suffer from painful intercourse and also frequent urinary tract infections.

Goldstein and associates address the issues of vaginal atrophy, its pathophysiology, and its resulting impact on female sexual health and function. Vaginal dryness not only occurs in mature women who have undergone menopause. Women who breast-feed, those who take certain medications, and those who suffer from a variety of other medical conditions can all suffer from vaginal dryness. Vaginal dryness can lead to painful intercourse, which then leads to avoidant behavior and results in lowered interest.

Women who suffer from atrophy should have an appropriate physical examination by a trained specialist. Vaginal atrophy and dryness is relatively easy to diagnose both by history and physical examination. Women complain of pain, irritation, discomfort in the vulva and vagina, and are fearful of pelvic and digital examinations. Sometimes, after detailed questioning, women often relay additional sexual complaints such as painful intercourse, lowered libido, and increased urinary tract infections. On clinical physical examination, the vagina is dry, pale, frail, and lacks the normal ridges and folds, elasticity, and pliability of a healthy vagina. There is minimal lubrication and the tissues are easily traumatized with pelvic examination. There can be petechiae, or small hemorrhages on the lining.

There are many choices for therapy, ranging from using vaginal moisturizers and lubricants to minimally absorbed vaginal estrogens. Replens or vitamin E can be applied to the vaginal area and can help hydrate the vaginal tissues. Lubricants without flavors, colors, and warming additives can and should be used during intercourse. Products such as petroleum jelly, extra virgin olive oil, and other household products should be avoided because they can change the natural balance of vaginal bacteria. If you are shy or perhaps embarrassed about purchasing lubrication products at a local store, try Drugstore.com, which offers discrete packaging and won't fill your inbox with loads of spam.

Sexual Pharmacology

Local treatment options for vaginal atrophy, where the product is placed within the vaginal area, include the use of local vaginal estrogens. They come in a variety of preparations including creams, rings, and tablets. The 17 beta estradiol tablets (Vagifem by NovoNordisk Pharmaceuticals) is an excellent choice for intravaginal dryness; it is safe, convenient, and well tolerated by women who are active. New lower doses should soon be available and show same efficacy. Creams, like Premarin Vaginal cream are also helpful for vulvovaginal dryness and discomfort, and this cream has an approved indication for this condition. Many women find introital discomfort troublesome, and these estrogen creams can be soothing and reverse symtomatolgy. This product as well will have some recent data published on new lower doses and minimal absorption profiles. The author has also recently published a small case series in the *Journal of Sexual Medicine* on the use of Premarin Vaginal cream as a potential orgasmic enhancer when rubbed directly into the clitoral tissue.

Although there is no one correct answer for how long you should or could remain on these products, clinically as long as you have symptoms and impaired quality of life or distress as a result of the complaints, treatment should continue. Interestingly, the North American Menopause Society (NAMS) discusses special populations including women who have had a malignancy and recommends that those without hormonally sensitive tumors be treated similarly to those who have vaginal atrophy with routine management. However, for those with hormonally sensitive tumors, such as breast carcinoma or endometrial cancer, treatment should be individualized and extensively discussed with their oncology and management teams.

You and your healthcare provider should discuss treatment options based on your preferences and his or her clinical expertise. Presently, adding a progestogen to the minimally absorbed local vaginal estrogen products is not warranted, and there is not enough data to support annual endometrial sampling or transvaginal ultrasound in women without symptoms.

Women's healthcare advocates often call vaginal dryness and its symptoms the silent epidemic because women are living longer. Because women are expected to live about one-third of their lives in menopause, quality-of-life concerns become paramount.

58. What are estrogen creams?

Premarin and Estrace cream are cream preparations containing conjugated estrogens that may be used for the vagina and vulvar tissues. These products come in a tube and often have plastic applicators to help with insertion. Many women find these products especially soothing to the irritated pelvic area. They have the added benefit that they can be tailored and managed individually using more or less of the product depending on your clinical situation.

The vulvar area, which is sensitive to estrogen levels, can become irritated and bothersome when hormonal levels are lowered. Women find estrogen creams especially comforting because they can be applied to the external pelvic area as well. The usual dosage is 2 to 4g (marked on the applicator) daily for 1 or 2 weeks, and then it is gradually reduced to one-half the initial dosage for a similar period. A maintenance dosage of approximately 1g can be used one to three times a week. It may be used after restoration of the vaginal lining has been achieved. You can attempt to discontinue or taper the medication during period of 3 to 6 months. Of course, if you experience any side effects or symptoms of vaginal bleeding while on the cream, you should speak with your healthcare provider. Newer lower doses have also been shown to be effective.

The food and drug administration has recently approved Duramed's (a subsidiary of Barr Pharmaceutical) synthetic, conjugated estrogen cream. It is a plant-derived local estrogen product that can be used for moderate to severe vaginal dryness and/or painful intercourse, both of which are symptoms of vulvar and vaginal atrophy often associated with the menopause.

The vulvar area, which is sensitive to estrogen levels, can become irritated and bothersome when hormonal levels are lowered.

Sexual Pharmacology

An interesting new and exciting use for vaginal estrogen creams is in the field of sexual arousal and orgasms. Recently, I published a small case series of women who used estrogen cream applied to the clitoral tissue because of decreased arousal and increased time to achieve orgasm. These women experienced increased arousal and increased orgasmic intensity when they applied estrogen cream to the clitoris. It may be helpful for you to use cream in the clitoral region as well if you are suffering from clitoral atrophy or have changes in arousal or orgasm. Ask your healthcare professional today.

59. What are vaginal estradiol tablets and vaginal rings?

Intravaginal estrogens are applied to the vaginal tissues and many products are minimally absorbed. Some sexual health providers prefer to prescribe minimally absorbed local 17 beta estradiol tablets. Vaginally administered estrogens in small, topically applied doses can be well absorbed. Patients say that the tablets are also easy to use, sometimes less messy than cream preparations, and technically easier to insert than estrogen rings.

Sometimes vaginal estradiol rings are prescribed for older women who complain of vaginal dryness and painful penetration. It is important to note that not all vaginal estrogen rings are the same and that they vary with respect to absorption into systemic circulation. Many women find them convenient because the rings are placed within the vaginal vault and are not changed for several months. The lower-dose vaginal rings release 7.5 micrograms per day of estradiol; this dose produces a steady state of serum (blood) levels of 6–8 pg/mL. This dose can treat local complaints of vaginal dryness but is not sufficient to treat hot flashes or other menopausal symptoms.

According to the North American Menopause Society's recent position statement concerning local vaginal estrogens, rings may change position during bowel movements, douching, and intercourse; however, there is no need to remove the ring during intercourse. In clinical experience, some women and men find rings uncomfortable. There are no data reporting on possible allergy to the silasitic plastic ring. Thickening of the endometrium or endometrial hyperplasia usually does not occur until levels surpass 19 pg/mL. The routine addition of a progestational agent is often not used and neither is it customary to recommend.

It is important to recognize that all estrogen products carry a black box warning and may mention some of the risks or complications. Some of the rare side effects include possible blood clots (thromboembolic events), increased heart problems (cardiovascular events), an increase in breast cancer, and increased endometrial cancer if unopposed with a progestin. The long-term safety data on minimally absorbed local vaginal estrogen products use in cancer patients remain to be further studied. Talk with your clinician to analyze which one may be the right solution for you and your partner.

60. What is testosterone replacement and how is it linked with women's sexuality?

Testosterone clearly has a role in sexual desire and overall female sexual function and should be considered as part of the complex and multifaceted treatment paradigm. However, replacement of testosterone in females remains controversial, and many researchers are still unconvinced about any direct linkage between testosterone and female sexual health. The data are confusing and conflicting. **Female androgen insufficiency syndrome** is considered a medical condition characterized by blunted or decreased motivation, persistent fatigue, and a decreased sense of personal well-being that is identified by sufficient plasma estrogen and low circulating bioavailability of testosterone as well as low sexual desire (libido). Other potential symptoms include bone loss, decreased muscle strength, and changes in cognition or memory. Bone density may also be affected.

Female androgen insufficiency syndrome

A constellation of symptoms attributed to low testosterone levels in women. Some of the symptoms include fatigue, decreased well-being, lack of energy or motivation, and decreased or absent sexual interest or desire.

Sexual Pharmacology

The North American Menopause Society published a comprehensive position statement in September 2005 that reviews testosterone use in women and includes monitoring, safety, and replacement guidelines and dosages for postmenopausal women. The society suggests that testosterone replacement may be helpful for certain postmenopausal women under certain circumstances (surgically menopausal or spontaneously menopausal). The position paper recommends testosterone in combination with estrogen replacement but also outlines clear follow-up guidelines and precautions that should be discussed with prospective patients. Informed consent and discussion of insufficient long-term safety data beyond 6 months is also required. This paper is crucial because to date there is no FDA-approved testosterone product for women, and many sexual medicine clinicians and healthcare providers are prescribing this medication (often off-label) to women.

A recent publication in the *New England Journal of Medicine*, "Testosterone for Low Libido in Post-Menopausal Women Not Taking Estrogen," showed that women who are not receiving estrogen treatment may have a modest and meaningful improvement in sexual function when they take the 300 microgram testosterone patch. There were more cases of breast cancer in the treatment arm of this study, and the researchers state that the long-term effects of testosterone on the breast remain uncertain.

At the time of publication of this book, there is no FDA-approved androgen product available for women. The use of male products or bioidentical products is off-label and should proceed with caution. More long-term safety data are warranted. It is interesting to note that in Europe a testosterone patch has recently been approved. It is now widely used in Europe, and many women in the United States and Canada are obtaining this medication over the Internet.

On the other hand, many healthcare providers are concerned about testosterone use because women are not ruled by testosterone or any other specific hormone. Dennerstein and associates from Australia present interesting data in an article titled "The Relative Effects of Hormones and Relationship Factors on Sexual Function of Women through the Natural Menopause Transition." The study was a prospective population-based questionnaire study of more than 300 Australian women that investigated the relative effects of hormonal and relationship factors on female sexual dysfunction during the natural menopausal transition. The results are provocative because they demonstrate that prior sexual functioning and relationship issues were more important than hormonal determinants of sexual function in midlife. Again, this is another supportive research article that reiterates that female sexual health is a complex interaction of hormones, biopsychosocial factors, and past sexual experiences.

Women are not victims of their hormones, and hormones, no matter the combination, are not the simple answer to sexual complaints. If you are unhappy because of poor communication with your partner and you're not sexually excited by your partner anymore, estrogen, progesterone, and testosterone may not change this situation. Hormones are often considered the mainstay of treatment for sexual complaints in woman and often they do help; however, to take them without looking at yourself as a total woman, your relationships with your partner, the dynamics in your household, and the psychostressors that influence your day-to-day activities is to miss the sexual health boat.

Very high levels of testosterone in products may have several potential serious side effects including, but not limited to, increased facial and body hair growth (hirsutism), weight gain, abnormal enlargement of the clitoris (clitoromegaly), hair loss (alopecia), changes in lipid profiles, and liver or hematologic changes. Women who have taken testosterone supplements have also have reported emotional changes. The safety of androgen in the cancer population has not been adequately studied. There is a concern that testosterone can be converted or aromatized to estrogen, which may reactivate, promote, or stimulate tumor growth. Long-term data on breast cancer risk is forthcoming and should be monitored. The new testosterone transdermal matrix patch has proven to be promising for female desire or libido issues; further randomized controlled trials that examine long-term safety are warranted. There is no silver bullet, and testosterone is not the sole answer to a complicated medical condition.

61. What are some common testosterone products?

Intrinsa, the only testosterone transdermal patch designed for women, is presently available in Europe for the treatment of hypoactive sexual desire disorder; however, it did not gain FDA approval in the United States. Many studies have been performed both locally and nationally. Many women are enjoying rekindled desire by using this product. It is a patch that is placed on the skin avoiding the first-pass mechanism of the liver and thereby minimizing some of the troublesome side effects.

Some of the other testosterones successfully used in women include oral methyl testosterone, transdermal testosterone, topical testosterone propionate cream 2%, testosterone gel, and oral dehydroepiandrosterone (DHEA). There are also medications that combine estrogen and an androgen component (Estratest and Estratest HS). Estratest is typically prescribed for refractory menopausal hot flashes that are not amenable to conventional estrogen replacement treatment.

Testopel is the only FDA-approved implantable cylindrical-shaped testosterone pellet that can be placed in the buttocks as a simple outpatient procedure. Testopels (testosterone pellets) have been used with success in male patients who have hypogonadism or testicular dysfunction. The product has also been used off-label for women with success for the treatment of lowered libido. Three pellets twice yearly can be implanted. Monitoring of serum levels is also needed. If side effects do occur, the implant can be removed as well with ease. A minor in-office procedure can place the pellets, and complications are minimal. Results are promising for improvement in libido.

Libigel is another testosterone product that is presently in stage 3 clinical trials. There are large ongoing trials looking at cardiovascular risk and breast cancer concerns with this new and innovative product. It is a gel that contains testosterone and can be applied to the upper arm. It has shown excellent, promising results for the treatment of hypoactive sexual desire disorder in menopausal women who have had a hysterectomy and are on a stable dose of estrogen. More data and studies should be forthcoming soon.

Testim is an FDA-approved product of testosterone replacement for men that can also be used off-label for women.

It is clear that women who decide to embark on testosterone treatment and who take testosterone off-label in an effort to have increased desire and libido should be under the care of a sexual medicine specialist. You need to have your blood laboratory values monitored closely. Your blood, lipids, and liver should be monitored and any side effects reported immediately to your clinician. If you experience any side effects, the medication should be adjusted. Return of libido should be monitored and you should be monitored for both breast health (mammograms) and cardiovascular health.

62. How can phosphodiesterase inhibitors (medications such as sildenafil [Viagra], tadalafil [Cialis], and vardenafil [Levitra]) be helpful to women? I thought they were only for men.

Phosphodiesterase inhibitors are medications that have been used in women for the treatment of sexual complaints. Phosphodiesterase inhibitors have been approved for the treatment of **erectile dysfunction** in men. Numerous attempts have

Erectile dysfunction

A persistent or recurrent inability to achieve or maintain an erection sufficient enough to accomplish a desired sexual behavior such as intercourse or coitus; earlier it was described as impotence.

been made to show an efficacy in women, but most fail to show any significant benefit in randomized clinical trials. The proposed mechanism of action is that the medication relaxes the clitoral and vaginal smooth muscle. Some potential side effects include headache, uterine contractions, dizziness, hypotension, myocardial infarction (heart attack), stroke, and sudden death. New and exciting emerging data may support their use in women who suffer from sexual complaints as a result of hypertension, diabetes, neural and vascular disease, or selective serotonin reuptake inhibitor (SSRI) use.

Recent data suggest that men who use phosphodiesterase inhibitors may actually be helping their spouses achieve sexual satisfaction. In a recent article titled "Through the Eyes of Women: The Partners' Perspective on Tadalafil," which was published in the *Journal of Urology* in September 2006, Althof and associates attempted to evaluate patient and partner responses to the efficacy and overall satisfaction with use of tadalafil to treat erectile dysfunction. This was a double-blinded placebo controlled 12-week trial of approximately 746 couples, who either received placebo or 10 mg or 20 mg of tadalafil. Female partners of men who were taking the medication reported significantly improved overall sexual satisfaction and corroborated the man's report of erectile improvement and penetration ability. The men were understandably happy and many reported improved erection, penetration, and overall satisfaction with the sexual experience while taking the medication. This study is one of many that examine the couple's response and receptiveness to treatment for erectile dysfunction. It is important to recognize that sexual complaints do not exist in an individual vacuum but rather intricately involve the partner and his or her reaction to treatment.

Treating one partner without examining the other is like assembling only half of a jigsaw puzzle.

Treating one partner without examining the other is like assembling only half of a jigsaw puzzle—you may get the fuzzy concept of the picture, but the clear, detailed picture is far from apparent. The concept is that sexual complaints, assessment, treatment, and compliance with therapeutics involve the dyad, the two individuals involved in the intimate relationship. To ignore the sexual partner may limit success in a treatment for a sexual health concern.

63. What is alprostadil cream?

Alprostadil cream is a prostaglandin E_1 cream that has been used in the past in men for the treatment of erectile dysfunction, but is not FDA-approved for the treatment of female sexual dysfunction. However, this topical medication in the form of a compounded cream can be applied to the pelvic genital area twice a day in women and acts assumedly by relaxing arterial smooth blood vessels, causing vasodilatation and increased sensitivity and sexual arousal. NexMed pharmaceutical company is conducting advanced randomized clinical trials with this cream with the intention of making it widely available in the United States sometime in the near future under the brand name Femprox.

A similar product is under investigation by Vivus under the name of Alista. There have been some stage 2 clinical trials. In a double-blind trial, 400 women with Female Sexual Arousal Disorder (FSAD) aged 21 to 65 years were randomized to receive a 10-dose at-home treatment of 500, 700, or 900 µg of alprostadil cream or a placebo cream. They were instructed to apply the cream to their clitoris and G-spot. More than 370 patients completed the study, and many showed significant improvement in sexual arousal. Possible side effects include pain to the genitals (which was decreased as the cream was washed away), lowered blood pressure, and possible temporary fainting (syncope). Alprostadil cream should be topically applied approximately 15 minutes before engaging in intercourse.

64. What is apomorphine?

Apomorphine is a medication that has been used sublingually for the treatment of male sexual health concerns. It is sometimes considered an alternative to the phosphodiesterase inhibitors. In a recent *Journal of Sexual Medicine* article, Bechara and associates published an excellent although small study titled "A Double-Blind Randomized Placebo Control Study Comparing the Objective and Subjective Changes in Female Sexual Response Using Sublingual Apomorphine." This small study attempted to show the effect of 3 mg of apomorphine with respect to subjective or objective changes in the female response cycle in those women who were diagnosed with orgasmic problems and those having difficulty reaching orgasm.

This study demonstrates that clitoral blood flow changes in peak velocity were significantly higher in the subjects who took the medication, which theoretically translates into better pelvic blood flow. This phenomenon, when considered in a broader light, would mean changes in arousal and lubrication. These areas were also significantly improved in the apomorphine group.

The researchers concluded that this medication was beneficial for women with orgasmic problems or difficulties in the domains of subjective and objective complaints. They also propose an anatomic mechanistic model of the function and result of the drug. The side effects and adverse events were low in incidence and mostly mild and also transient. Although this study had very small numbers, many sexual healthcare professionals are optimistic because the medication is provocative and warrants further rigorous study for the treatment of female sexual complaints. It is presently not available for prescription to female sexual health patients, but studies are ongoing.

65. How can the antidepressant bupropion (Wellbutrin) be helpful to my sexual health?

Bupropion is a nonserotonin reuptake inhibitor antidepressant dopamine agonist that has recently been touted as the medication for depression treatment with the least sexual side effects. This medication is a weak blocker of the uptake of the brain chemicals serotonin and norepinephrine and is commonly used in smoking-cessation programs. A typical trial of this medication includes a starting dose of 75 mg that can be increased gradually. Precautions and possible side effects include insomnia, nervousness, and mild to moderate increases in blood pressure as well as a risk of lowering seizure threshold.

Seagraves and Dr. Anita Clayton published a study titled "Bupropion Sustained Release for the Treatment of Hypoactive Sexual Desire in Premenopausal Women" in the *Journal of Clinical Psychopharmacology*. This was a landmark study that examined women with idiopathic acquired or global hypoactive sexual desire disorder in a randomized placebo controlled trial with escalating dose of bupropion. All measures indicated increased sexual responsiveness, and changes in the Sexual Function Questionnaire demonstrated increased sexual arousal, orgasmic completion, and sexual satisfaction. The researchers propose a mechanism by which the medication operates and causes positive sexual effects by acting on the dopamine and norepinephrine pathways. The concepts that this medication acted centrally or in the brain were reinforced, and it did improve sexual functioning and desire in many women.

There are minimal side effects, and most women can tolerate this medication. It has been used extensively by sexual medicine healthcare providers off-label for complaints of low desire. It is also used in breast cancer patients who suffer from lowered libido. This already FDA-approved medication (for another indication), which acts centrally, warrants further detailed study as a possible treatment for sexual desire complaints in women.

66. What is Flibanserin?

Flibanserin is a 5-HT1A agonist/5-HT2 antagonist. It is manufactured by a private German company called Boehringer Ingelheim and was initially produced as an antidepressant medication. In the late 1990s, the company had developed a molecule called flibanserin that seemed to relieve

Sexual Pharmacology

stress in rats. But unfortunately this medication flopped for this indication. It has a half-life of approximately 7 hours and appears to be safe with minimal interactions with other medications.

Flibanserin shows excellent promise for treatment of hypoactive sexual desire disorder in women. The medication is now in stage 3 clinical trials, and many sexual healthcare providers assume effectiveness with minimal side effect profiles. Most sexual healthcare providers are elated because this medication is not a hormone. It acts centrally and some of the side effects include nausea, dizziness, fatigue, sleeplessness, increased bleeding if on a nonsteroidal anti-inflammatory drug or aspirin. It is perhaps the most promising medication pending for the treatment of female sexual desire disorder. Unfortunately, it is not yet clear exactly how flibanserin works. The company researchers have figured out that it affects several circuits in the brain that may be linked to feelings of enjoyment and pleasure. It may act as a serotonin modulator that restores the balance of this compound. It may restore hormonal balance.

According to the company's spokesperson, one of those brain circuits apparently helps control sexual desire and arousal. The effects of the drugs are not immediate and may take some time to take effect. Recently, data from the Rose study, an open label randomized withdrawal study, were presented in Europe and demonstrated increased desire days and increased satisfying sexual events for women on this medication. Adverse events were minimal, and women who abruptly stopped this medication did not suffer from acute withdrawal syndromes.

Boehringer Ingelheim has placed a large investment in this medication. The company has launched four major clinical trials, involving 5000 women in 220 worldwide locations, with the goal of applying for Food and Drug Administration approval in 2009. Sexual healthcare providers are eagerly awaiting the news of a potential treatment for female hypoactive sexual desire disorder. Flibanserin was recently featured in *Business Week* magazine and gained publicity and notoriety for the most plausible treatment for hypoactive sexual desire disorder.

There is also a company-sponsored disease registry that will follow many women over the course of 2 years with serial questionnaires. The Southern California Center for Sexual Health and Survivorship Medicine was chosen as a premier vanguard site. Eligible participants may enroll after the informed consent procedure and are entitled to remuneration.

67. What is tibolone?

Tibolone (Livial) is a synthetic hormone-type drug. It is used mainly for hormone replacement therapy in post-menopausal women. Tibolone can help relieve symptoms of the menopause transition including hot flashes, night sweats, mood changes, and vaginal dryness and vaginal irritation. It can also help to prevent bone health issues such as osteoporosis (a loss of bone mass so that bones become brittle and easily broken).

Generic tibolone tablets are not yet available. Many studies over the last 5 years show that tibolone, a new female hormone, shares many effects with male hormones and may help to prevent bone problems and lack of sexual desire. It does not increase breast cancer risk and does not have to be taken with progesterone to prevent uterine cancer. Tibolone's cardiovascular effects are much more murky. On the positive side, the drug reduces total cholesterol and harmful triglycerides and slightly lowers low-density lipoproteins (LDLs, or bad cholesterol). But it also lowers high-density lipoproteins (HDL, or good cholesterol). Many experts are concerned about this mixed picture, and it may affect cardiovascular health.

Livial is available in much of continental Europe and in the United Kingdom, but is not yet available in the United States. Basically, this molecule combines some of the positive effects of estrogen, progesterone, and testosterone. It has been shown to reduce hot flashes, increase bone mineral density, and women report that it decreases vaginal dryness. The drug does improve desire, but researchers are uncertain of its effect on other parameters of female sexual function. There are some medical concerns regarding the lipid metabolism, hemostasis, and long-term cardiovascular and cancer risks.

68. What is Bremelanotide?

PT-141 (Bremelanotide) is a melanocortin receptor agonist that is under study and development for the treatment of female sexual complaints. It is also used in the treatment of male sexual complaints. Originally, this medication was developed and tested as a sunless tanning agent but did not induce the desired effects; however, it was noticed that some subjects reported increased sexual arousal and spontaneous erections. Some serious concerns regarding the benefit and risk ratio of Bremelanotide caused delay in the stage 3 clinical trial regarding some severe changes in blood pressure. The melanocortins are thought to play an important role in female sexual health and functioning. The medication, which is under study and in advanced clinical trials, is a centrally acting drug that can affect the brain. It is a colorless, odorless chemical that is placed within a nasal inhaler and has been used by many women with sexual complaints. Some women who have taken the medication have reported increased warmth or throbbing in the genitals as well as an associated increased desire to engage in intercourse after use of the drug in pilot studies. A phase 2A pilot clinical study looked at this medication in premenopausal women diagnosed with female sexual dysfunction (FSD) and it has not shown encouraging results.

On May 13, 2008, Palatin Technologies, the maker of Bremelanotide, announced it has discontinued further development of Bremelanotide for the treatment of both male and female sexual dysfunction. However, the company released a statement identifying that it is also advancing a new compound, PL-6983, which in animal models causes significantly lower increases in blood pressure than those seen with Bremela-notide, into phase 1 clinical studies for treatment of male and female sexual dysfunction. There is hope in the future, and we should await further studies and publications.

69. What are vaginal moisturizers?

The liberal use of local nonmedicated, nonhormonal vaginal moisturizers such as Replens or vitamin E suppositories can provide relief for the symptoms of vaginal atrophy. These agents are recommended for use two or three times weekly. Women should wear a light pad when using vitamin E suppositories because they may stain undergarments. They help improve the vaginal lining or mucosa and help maintain the ridges and folds within the vaginal tissues. They should be used independently of sexual intercourse. Other types of moisturizers claim to be all natural. Another option is Moist Again. KY Vaginal liquid beads (Johnson and Johnson) are also another excellent vaginal moisturizer. KY Silk E (Johnson and Johnson) is also a popular vaginal moisturizer as is Vagisil.

As the number one recommended product, Replens (Lil' Drugstore Products) has been leading the way to increase the visibility of vaginal moisturizers among women seeking alternatives to hormone therapy. In past years, the *New England Journal of Medicine* reported that Replens was just as effective at relieving vaginal dryness as prescription hormones. Over-the-counter, Replens Vaginal Moisturizer provides soothing, immediate, and long-lasting relief from feminine dryness for 72 hours. Replens is available over-the-counter in many local pharmacies. In a published randomized trial, a polycarbophil-based vaginal moisturizer that is available over the counter (Replens) provided relief of vaginal (dryness) symptoms.

70. What are vaginal lubricants?

Vaginal lubricants are products that you can purchase over-the-counter that can be placed in the vagina before sexual activity to help create a sense of moisture or lubrication. Some

The liberal use of local nonmedicated, nonhormonal vaginal moisturizers such as Replens or vitamin E suppositories can provide relief for the symptoms of vaginal atrophy.

Sexual Pharmacology

women have decreased natural ability to create lubrication on their own, so store-bought or commercially available lubricants can be used to maintain a moist environment so that intercourse is not painful. The use of water-based vaginal lubricants with intercourse is also encouraged when vaginal dryness and atrophy are diagnosed.

Not all lubricants are created equal. Vaginal lubricants that contain spermicides, bactericides, perfumes, coloration, and flavors may also irritate a sensitive vaginal lining. Warming additives and fruit flavors may contain chemical irritants as well. These additives can be problematic especially in menopausal women. Read the labels because you can develop sensitivities to some of the chemicals in lubricants. Some of the common offenders include glycerin and parabens.

Lubricants can be purchased online discreetly, and many are available in your local pharmacy. Lubricate all surfaces as part of foreplay and be sure to keep lubricant handy in case more is needed. Lubricants may be water- or silicone-based. The lubricants come in a variety of different textures and viscosities; experiment with different types to find the type that is best for you. There are many different brands with different qualities. Some are warming, some are not. Some formulations do not contain glycerin or parabens. Some types are both fragrance-free and latex-compatible and can be used to increase your and your partner's sensual sensitivity and for total-body massage.

PART SEVEN

Alternative and Complementary Medicine and Sexuality

What are pheromones and how can scent affect
sexuality?

Can certain foods enhance sexuality?

Can exercise be used to improve sexual function?

More . . .

From the beginning of time, civilizations have been seeking alternative methods to enhance and improve sexuality and sexual performance. It is rumored that as she sailed down the Nile, Cleopatra soaked the sails of her boat in ylang-ylang, an aromatic essential oil supposedly used for sexual attractiveness, to attract and excite the famed Mark Antony. Sexual mythology also suggests that the sensual playboy Casanova ate chocolate oysters before his sexual escapades. It is also believed that ancient Romans and Greeks consumed figs before their sexual orgies because those foods were believed to contain essential minerals needed to produce sex hormones.

According to the *Cambridge History of Food*, "Aphrodisiacs were first sought out as a remedy for various sexual anxieties including fears of inadequate performance as well as a need to increase fertility." The term **aphrodisiac** has Greek roots: *aphrodisiakos*, from *aphrodisiac*, meaning sexual pleasures. In Greek mythology, Aphrodite was the goddess of love, beauty, sensuality, and sex. A more global definition of *aphrodisiac* is foods, scents, beverages, drinks, mineral supplements, or chemicals that are believed to increase or enhance sexual desire, performance, or stamina. The human quest for sexual enhancers or natural substances is as old as the legendary quest for the Holy Grail.

Women and men continue to try many unconventional sexual enhancers and therapeutics to facilitate treatment for sexual function complaints and arousal disorders. There are limited scientifically proven databases containing results of randomized control trial studies that demonstrate beneficial use of these methods for alleviating sexual dysfunction. In fact, many have some concerning side effects and can interact with prescription medications. It is always best to consult with your physician as to whether a particular product is right for you. This section highlights a few of the more frequently used products.

Aphrodisiac

A substance believed to improve or enhance sexual function or pleasure. Some think it may stimulate feelings of love, intimacy, or desire.

The human quest for sexual enhancers or natural substances is as old as the legendary quest for the Holy Grail.

---

71. How can herbs affect sexuality?

Many herbal supplements are marketed as having sensuality- and sexuality-enhancing properties. Some of the more popular ones are described in the following subsections.

Yohimbine

Yohimbine is an herb that is prevalent in West Africa. It has been used as an aphrodisiac. It is also combined with supplements in formulas to improve athletic prowess and is believed to treat both male and female sexual dysfunction. The active component, an alkaloid called yohimbine, has been used in clinical studies for erectile difficulties in men. There is no conclusive evidence that this product is effective for the treatment of female sexual complaints; however, it does stimulate the central nervous system and also acts as a monoamine oxidase inhibitor and calcium channel blocker. Caution should be exercised because it can potentially interact with numerous drugs, causing severe adverse effects.

DHEA

DHEA is the most abundant hormone secreted by the adrenal glands. It is used to enhance sexual performance, prevent atherosclerosis, and stimulate the immune system. It circulates in the blood as the sulfate ester, dehydroepiandrosterone-3-sulfate (DHEA-S), which is a precursor for other hormones, including estrogen and androgens. It has been shown to alter some of the activities of the cytochrome P-450 enzyme that metabolizes a number of drugs. Taking DHEA can elevate your estrogen level as well as your testosterone levels. Too much DHEA can cause serious side effects, and if you do choose to begin this supplement, be certain to understand your risks and be under the direct supervision of a sexual medicine healthcare provider.

In premenopausal women, high levels of DHEA have been associated with increased ovarian and breast cancer risk. High DHEA-S levels have also been shown to contribute to

Yohimbine

An alkaloid medicine derived from the South American plant *Corynanthe yohimbe*, which has alleged aphrodisiac properties.

Alternative and Complementary Medicine and Sexuality

121

tamoxifen resistance and disease progression in breast cancer. Unfortunately, there have been limited well-designed randomized control trials that provide evidence to support use of DHEA for the treatment of sexual complaints.

Maca

Maca is a native Peruvian plant used in traditional medicine for strength and to enhance fertility. It is believed to help in sexual behavior in both men and women, and may be used in attempts to relieve menopausal symptoms. Maca was shown in animal studies to increase sexual function. Despite some of the medical literature, there is still insufficiently strong medical evidence to support of the use of maca for female sexual dysfunction. The therapeutic dose and toxicity of maca are unknown.

Wild Yam

Wild yam is derived from the root of a twining vine. Wild yam was traditionally thought to have antispasmodic properties and was promoted for gastrointestinal and menstrual dysfunction. Diosgenin, a chemical component found in wild yam, has been shown to have estrogenic and progestogenic effects in mice; however, there is no scientific evidence that this substance can be converted by the body into human hormones. Some wild yam extract creams have been marketed as a natural source of progesterone, although they contain synthetic progesterone that is not connected to wild yam. There is no evidence of its efficacy in alleviating sexual dysfunction.

Chaste Berry

Chaste berry is derived from the fruit of the chaste berry tree and contains steroidal precursors and active moieties including progesterone, testosterone, and androstenedione. Clinical studies suggest that in women it is efficacious in reducing symptoms associated with PMS, but there is no evidence to prove its effectiveness for sexual complaints. Chaste berry may interact with oral contraceptives, other hormonal therapy, and dopamine antagonists (such as haloperidol and prochlorpera-zine). Some of the common reported adverse effects include nausea, rash, headache, and agitation.

Horny Goat Weed

Horny goat weed, or *Epimedium*, is a Chinese herb used in traditional medicine to treat fatigue, arthritic and nerve pain, and sexual dysfunction. It is also known as Yin Yang Huo in Chinese medicine. However, there is no clinical evidence to support the use of *Epimedium* for sexual dysfunction. There is some evidence to support the fact that extended used can cause dizziness, nosebleeds, and thirst.

Ginseng

Ginseng is derived from the root of the ginseng plant and is used to improve athletic performance, strength, and stamina. It is also used as an immunostimulant for people with dia-betes, cancer, HIV/AIDS, and a variety of other conditions. However, a systematic review of clinical trials on ginseng found no evidence of its efficacy for any of these indications. It has been promoted in the treatment of erectile dysfunction, but current studies to support this claim are limited.

72. What are some combination products?

ArginMax is a combination of 13 essential vitamins and nu-trients that has been studied at the University of Stanford, University of Hawaii, and Albany Medical College. It is a nutritional supplement composed of *Gingko biloba*, Panax ginseng, American ginseng, damiana, L-arginine, vitamins A, C, E, B-complex, zinc, and selenium. It is being promoted to help both female sexual dysfunction and erectile dysfunction in men. L-arginine, a major component of the product, may adversely affect asthmatics, so caution should be exercised in this patient group. A small pilot study demonstrated im-provement in a variety of sexual domains, including sexual satisfaction, arousal, and desire in women who suffered with sexual dysfunction and in men with erectile dysfunction. Men reported overall improvement in ability to maintain an erection during intercourse and overall improvement in sexual fitness and satisfaction. This product contains ginseng that was shown to have possible estrogenic effects, but other studies did not corroborate this possibility.

Avlimil is considered a dietary supplement that is being promoted to help alleviate symptoms associated with female sexual dysfunction and lowered desire. It consists of sage leaf, red raspberry leaf, kudzu root extract, red clover extract, capsicum pepper, licorice root, bayberry fruit, damiana leaf, valerian root, ginger root, and black cohosh root. Avlimil is thought to enhance sexual satisfaction by increasing blood flow and by promoting muscle relaxation. A small unpublished clinical trial involving 49 women found Avlimil to have a positive effect on sexual response. Researchers mentioned that there were significant changes toward a positive improvement in desire, arousal, and orgasm. There are minimal side effects, which can include minor stomach upset and minor irritation. Some of the ingredients such as sage, kudzu, red clover, and black cohosh may have estrogenic actions and may interfere with tamoxifen. Caution should be exercised if you have a hormonally dependent tumor. However, the ingredients in the commercial product are different from those used in the study.

Xzite is an herbal combination product of *Acanthopanax*, *Ligusticum wallichi*, and *Chrysanthemum morbifolium* and is being marketed as a female sexual enhancer. According to a small unpublished study, Xzite was more effective than a placebo in increasing female sexual pleasure. The mechanism of action is not known. No adverse effects have been reported from use of Xzite.

Libidol is a nutritional supplement used for female sexual dysfunction. It consists of a combination of sage leaf, red raspberry leaf, kudzu root extract, red clover extract, bayberry fruit, capsicum pepper, damiana leaf, ginger root, licorice root, valerian root, black cohosh root, essential amino acid, horny goat weed, wild oats, niacin, L-arginine, and DHEA. The herbal components are thought to relieve symptoms of sexual dysfunction in women. There is no scientific evidence to support use of Libidol.

73. What is feminine arousal fluid?

Feminine arousal fluid (Zestra) is a topical botanical formulation of borage seed oil, evening of primrose oil, angelica root extract, *Coleus forskohlii* extract, ascorbyl palmitate, and alpha tocopherol, and it shows promise as a topical formulation for sexual enhancement. The author's clinical experience finds Zestra helps many women achieve sexual wellness, increased arousal, and overall sexual and sensual satisfaction. The use of feminine arousal fluid results in increased clitoral and vaginal warmth, heightened arousal, and increased sexual pleasure in selected women. A small clinical trial involving 20 women showed that Zestra benefits both normal women and those with female sexual arousal disorder. Zestra was also noted to be helpful in women on antidepressants such as serotonin reuptake inhibitors (SSRIs). Caution should be exercised when using this oil when you have dryness or atrophic tissues. Some women report increased irritation or burning after application. The oil can be rubbed into the clitoral tissues prior to self-stimulation or intercourse.

The use of feminine arousal fluid results in increased clitoral and vaginal warmth, heightened arousal, and increased sexual pleasure in selected women.

Some healthcare providers also use feminine arousal fluids in the sexual rehabilitation of cervical cancer patients who have lowered sensation in the genital pelvic area. More clinical research is needed to prove its usefulness; however, patients subjectively report improved arousal and sensation after radiation or trauma. Larger clinical trials are in the process of being completed.

74. What is an intimacy-enhancing cream?

Intimacy-enhancing topical creams (for example, Escalate) are designed for women to use to help sensitize their clitorises. The products contain L-arginine (an amino acid essential for the production of nitric oxide), which can create an invigorating sensation when applied to the clitoral tissues. These creams have also been known to create a stimulating sensation for men, too. The amino acid L-arginine enhances female sexual response by stimulating the increase of blood flow to the clitoris.

For some women using a cream, orgasm will occur with increased frequency or intensity. In research studies performed by one manufacturer of an intimacy-enhancing cream, about 80% of the women found that the cream extended their natural orgasms and improved responses through three or more successive uses. Creams are supplied in airless pump bottles that provide approximately 30 applications. There are no known side effects and creams are manufactured under the guidance of the GMP standards (Good Manufacturing Practices). Escalate is helpful for women on multiple medications because it does not interfere with any medication. Place a small amount (half a pump) of cream on your fingertips and apply it to the underside of your clitoris and rub thoroughly for several minutes. Almost immediately, you will feel an invigorating warm sensation.

Blood circulation may increase and tissues will become considerably more sensitive. You may reapply after a few minutes if desired. The sensations may last for about 20 to 30 minutes and creams are completely safe for ingestion; some have a pleasant cinnamon fragrance and taste, which can be pleasurable for some men. Some men also report increased invigorating sensations with cream use. If irritation occurs or if you are nursing or pregnant, you should not use the product. Johnson and Johnson is investigating another interesting product, PD-F 5394, which is a nonhormonal over-the-counter female arousal gel for sexual enhancement. Preliminary studies presented at a recent educational seminar demonstrated that the gel enhanced the sexual experience of healthy women with adequate sexual functioning; it improves sexual arousal and lubrication and it is well tolerated with minimal adverse effects or genital irritation. Another study reported that in home use of the female arousal gel applied to the clitoris, it was associated with enhanced sexual arousal, orgasmic intensity, sexual satisfaction, and pleasure. Release of this new product is slated for sometime in 2009.

75. What are pheromones and how can scent affect sexuality?

Pheromones are chemicals substances excreted by an organism that elicit behavioral responses from another like species member. When humans experience a scent, it often produces an emotional response based upon an associated memory. Research scientists have found that inhaling an odor can modify brain waves, and it is believed that the scent is perceived by one's learned memory in the amygdala, which is a part of the limbic system (the emotional center of the brain). This system also controls emotions related to fear, aggression, stress, anxiety, and sexuality. **Aromatherapy** is the use of essential oils distilled from aromatic plants for therapeutic purposes. The aromas of ylang-ylang and jasmine have been traditionally used to increase sexuality. A recent study found that the scent of cinnamon may also increase sexual desire through an unknown mechanism.

Female sexual pheromones have been shown to attract mates of the opposite sex in insects, rodents, and seals. In some organisms, these chemicals also can reveal identity and stimulate **ovulation**, or egg production, and sexual development. Humans have historically been thought to have advanced eye/optical and verbal systems but only a moderate olfactory system; therefore, the presence of pheromones in humans and its sociosexual effect has only recently been addressed. The organ that detects sex pheromones in some animals is called the vomeronasal organ (VNO). A tiny, possibly nonfunctional VNO in humans has recently been found far within the inside of the nasal cavity, but whether this organ actually neurologically connects to the brain is unknown. Human pheromones are mostly produced in the apocrine glands that

Pheromone

A volatile compound released by one organism that triggers a specific behavior in another member of the same species.

When humans experience a scent, it often produces an emotional response based upon an associated memory.

Aromatherapy

An integrative care practice that uses oils from plants to treat physical or psychological conditions. The oils can be inhaled, used in vaporizers, or used in massage.

Ovulation

The process of egg release from the ovary.

Alternative and Complementary Medicine and Sexuality

are located in the axillae and pubic regions. They may also be found in other gland secretions such as urine, saliva, and sweat. The pheromones are produced only after puberty when mate selection begins, and their production decreases during the menopause transition.

In humans, chemicals released in sweat and other secretions may positively affect the mood of the opposite sex. Interestingly, humans often perceive the pheromone as odorless and their physiologic and behavioral response may be subconscious. Studies that examined topically applied synthesized human pheromones to **perimenopausal** women have shown to increase affectionate gestures such as hugging, kissing, and petting. When a researcher studied human pheromones in a laboratory, he also noted that they imparted a sense of warmth and friendliness among coworkers in the corporate setting.

Although the topical use of pheromones can increase sexual attraction, affection, pleasant moods, and confidence, there is no sound medical, evidence-based data to support the notion that pheromones may increase sexual activity. Modern social practices such as daily showering or bathing with soap, perfumes, antiperspirants, and use of birth control pills can reverse human's natural ability to perceive another's natural scent. Olfactory researchers say that natural human aromas or scents may play only a subtle part in the phenomenon of human attraction, and that psychosocial and cultural characteristics may play a larger part.

Researcher David Berliner produces scents (Realm for Men and Realm for Women) that include human pheromones. The manufacturer claims that pheromones of the opposite sex positively affect the person's mood and thus may cause the wearer to feel more attractive and confident. Although thought provoking, use of aromas and human pheromones have not been demonstrated with any degree of medical certainty to support the widely held belief that they may be associated with improved sexual vitality and function.

Perimenopause

The time in which women are having irregular periods before the periods completely stop. It can be several years in duration and is characterized by menopausal and nonmenopausal symptomatology.

76. Can certain foods enhance sexuality?

According to George Armelagos, PhD, virtually every culture has associated food with intimacy and sensuality, and practically every food at one time or another has been associated with sexual performance or improved functioning. Folklore claims that sesame seeds were considered the pearls of sexual nutrition that Cleopatra used to seduce Julius Caesar and Mark Antony. Tables 2 and 3 show the most popular foods and spices that are claimed to have sexual-enhancing properties. Most men and women still hold fast the notion that nutrition can treat or enhance sexual function despite the fact that there is no scientific data to support their usage.

Virtually every culture has associated food with intimacy and sensuality, and practically every food at one time or another has been associated with sexual performance or improved functioning.

Table 2   Aphrodisiacs: Foods

• Almonds	• Honey
• Anchovies	• Horseradish
• Artichokes	• Lettuce
• Arugula	• Lobster
• Asparagus	• Mangos
• Avocado	• Mussels
• Banana	• Onions
• Caffeine	• Oysters
• Carrots	• Radishes
• Caviar	• Salmon
• Champagne	• Scallops
• Cheese	• Strawberries
• Chocolate	• Tomatoes
• Coffee	• Truffles
• Eggs	• Wine
• Figs	• Yams
• Ginseng	

Table 3   Aphrodisiacs: Spices

• Basil	• Curry
• Cardamom	• Garlic
• Cayenne pepper	• Ginkgo biloba
• Chili pepper	• Licorice
• Cinnamon	• Nutmeg
• Clover	• Onions
• Coriander	• Vanilla
• Cumin	• Garlic

Alternative and Complementary Medicine and Sexuality

Seafood such as oysters, salmon, scallops, and sardines contain healthy monounsaturated fats called omega-3 fatty acids. Fish are also rich in zinc, which is an essential nutrient for testosterone production. Because the goddess Aphrodite was said to be born from the sea, many types of seafood have historically been believed to be aphrodisiacs. Oysters are particularly esteemed as sex aids because of their zinc content.

Honey is another favorite aphrodisiac and, according to folklore, newlyweds were supposed to have consumed "honey wine," which was thought to increase sexual stamina. It is thought that the word *honeymoon*, which was coined in ancient Europe, is derived from this concept. The ancient Egyptians believed in the stimulating properties of honey, which has an eternal quality to it. Honey is also believed to enhance one's sexual stamina by providing an immediate carbohydrate supply to boost lovers' energy. Honey is also thought to offset the effects of alcohol by slowing down the absorption of alcohol by the stomach.

Ginseng has been used as an invigorating and rejuvenating agent for centuries in China, Tibet, Korea, Indochina, and India. The root may have a mild stimulant action similar to coffee. Some experiments report a sexual response in animals treated with ginseng, but there is no evidence that ginseng has an effect on human sexuality. The word *ginseng* means "man root," and the plant's reputation as an aphrodisiac probably arises from its marked similarity in shape to the human body.

The similarity of the shape of the rhinoceros horn to the penis is credited for its worldwide reputation as a libido enhancer. The horn contains significant amounts of calcium and phosphorus, which are thought to improve general physical vigor and possibly lead to an increased sexual interest.

Spanish fly, or cantharides, is manufactured from dried beetle remains and is probably the most legendary food with aphrodisiac-like properties—and perhaps the most deadly. The reported sexual excitement from Spanish fly originates from the irritative effects on the urogenital tract and resultant rush of blood to the sex organs. However, the toxin can burn the mouth and throat and can lead to genitourinary infections, scarring of the urethra, and even death. The active ingredient of Spanish fly, cantharidin, can also cause kidney malfunction or gastrointestinal hemorrhages with excessive consumption.

77. Are sexual diets fact or fiction?

A sexual diet is basically a prescribed nutritional plan that advocates the benefits of general health maintenance to improve sexual performance and possibly treat sexual complaints. Most specialized diets claim that weight reduction and decreased depressive thoughts combined with improved immunity and release of natural endorphins will promote sexuality.

Several popular diets have been marketed directly to the public for improved sexual virility and function and are discussed in the following subsections. Exercise precaution when considering any of these diets because some of these aphrodisiac-like diets can be hazardous to your health.

It is important to note that none of the diets have been shown in randomized clinical trials to enhance, improve, or restore sexual function. According to an article written by Tamar Nordenberg (a lawyer with the Office of the Director in the FDA's Center for Drug Evaluation and Research), the "reputed sexual effects of so-called aphrodisiacs are based in folklore, not fact." In 1989, the FDA affirmed that there was no methodical scientific verification that any over-the-counter aphrodisiacs exerted any effect to treat sexual dysfunction.

The Mediterranean Diet

In a recent article published in the *Journal of Impotence Research*, Esposito and colleagues looked at the Mediterranean diet and showed that it did improve sexual function in women with metabolic syndrome (increased abdominal adiposity, low HDLs, hypertriglyceridemia, increased blood pressure, and abnormal glucose metabolism). The diet was regulated and consisted of whole grains, fruits, vegetables, legumes, walnuts, and olive oil. Those with metabolic syndrome were monitored closely, screened with the standard Female Sexual Function Index, and kept nutritional diaries. They were subject to intense follow-up. They were also noted to have lowered levels of C-reactive protein, a substance that may be implicated in vascular inflammation. They were advised to increase consumption of fish and decrease intake of red or processed meat. Both the diet and the placebo groups were advised to increase exercise levels mainly by walking, playing aerobic ball games, or swimming for a minimum of 30 minutes per day. The placebo group was given information concerning healthy food choices but no specific program was offered to them.

According to the American Heart Association, there is no one specific Mediterranean diet. At least 16 countries border the Mediterranean Sea and diets vary between countries. There are many differences in culture, ethnicity, religion, economy, and agriculture. Some dietary pattern that have emerged include the following:

- Many fruits, vegetables, bread and other cereals, potatoes, beans, nuts and seeds are consumed.
- Olive oil is an important monounsaturated fat source.
- Dairy products including yogurt, fish, and poultry are consumed in low to moderate amounts, and little red meat is eaten.
- Eggs are consumed zero to four times a week.
- Low amounts of full-fat cheeses are eaten.
- Wine is consumed in low to moderate amounts.
- Adequate hydration is key in this diet.

More than half the fat calories in a Mediterranean diet come from monounsaturated fats (mainly from olive oil). Monounsaturated fat doesn't raise blood cholesterol levels the way saturated fat does.

The Orgasmic Diet

The orgasmic diet consists of avoiding antidepressants, coffee, tea, caffeine, soft drinks, cigarettes, herbal stimulants, ginkgo, and ginseng while adding high-dose vitamins such as a multivitamin, vitamin E (400 IU), vitamin C, fish oil (6 g), calcium (100 mg), magnesium (400 mg), zinc (15 mg), and slow-release iron. This diet advocates maintaining a "Zone type" dietary balance of low carbohydrates, while including pelvic exercises called **Kegel exercises**. It also includes one ounce of dark chocolate.

The Testosterone Diet

The testosterone diet includes a variety of nuts, olive oil, canola oil, peanut butter, turnips, broccoli, cabbage, mustard greens, Brussels sprouts, collard greens, watercress, bok choy, and radishes. It advocates avoiding alcohol, getting adequate sleep, and exercising. The Gladiator Diet and the Testosterone Advantage Plan are other dietary plans that claim to enhance sexual virility and performance through weight lifting and eating a diet of 33% carbohydrates, 33% fats, and 33% protein while avoiding alcohol, sweets, and processed food. Other diets not only incorporate foods and nutrition, but also advocate sexual exercises that can be completed with your intimate partner.

Other Diets and Cookbooks

The Ultimate Sex Diet by Kerry McCloskey focuses on aphrodisiacs, whereas the *Great American Sex Diet* by Laura Corn recommends frequent sexual activity.

An interesting cookbook titled *The New InterCourses: An Aphrodisiac Cookbook* by Martha Hopkins and Randall Lockridge is devoted to recipes that use erotically charged ingredients and is directed to those who may be interested in incorporating sexual foods into their diet. It features interesting recipes such as Black Russian Cake, Pasta with Rosemary Cream Sauce, and Oysters with Chardonnay Wine. Another interesting book is

Kegel exercises
Exercises designed to increase muscle strength and elasticity in the pelvis. They may be recommended in the treatment of urinary incontinence.

called *Seduction and Spice* by Rudolf Sodamin. It is wonderful, exciting cookbook that combines recipes with sexual folklore, history, and aphrodisiac tales.

Chocolate and Sexuality?

Chocolate is by far the most popular food associated with sexuality.

Chocolate is by far the most popular food associated with sexuality. It is associated with romance, apology, and seductive gifts. The Aztecs referred to chocolate as nourishment of the Gods, and according to legend, the Aztec emperor Montezuma consumed 50 glasses of honey-sweetened chocolate to maintain his virility and potency before visiting his harem of more than 600 women. The 18th-century lover Casanova thought that chocolate was an aphrodisiac because eating it produces the same satisfying sensations as sex.

Chocolate does contain the biogenic amines tyramine and phenylethamine (PEA, the love drug), methylxanthines, and cannabinoid-like fatty acids. Cocoa is found in bitter chocolate and it may increase sensitivity. Fabbri and colleagues studied the concept that chocolate was an effective aphrodisiac that increased sexual desire and pleasure in women. As recently published in the *Journal of Sexual Medicine*, after controlling for age, there was no difference in changes in sexual function as measured by the Female Sexual Function Index of chocolate consumers versus nonconsumers. It is tempting to suppose that chocolate may have some positive effects on sexual function; however, it is not substantiated in the medical literature.

78. Can acupuncture help my libido?

Acupuncture and herbal Chinese medicine incorporate more than 2,000 years of experience in treating sexual dysfunction. Multiple studies have concluded that when acupuncture needles are placed in specific key locations of the body, many processes are activated including hormone release, nervous system regulation, and increased vascular blood flow. In addition to stimulating and regulating the physical body, acupuncture also has a profound calming effect on mental and emotional states, thus enhancing feelings of well-being and sexual desire.

Acupuncture has been used for several hundred years to treat a variety of medical concerns including pelvic pain, headaches, menopausal hot flashes, and anxiety. In my institution, we have developed an acupuncture and herbal medicine program that specifically addresses the concerns of women who are suffering from lowered libido. Our comprehensive approach couples both Eastern and Western medical practices, which have proven beneficial for women suffering from sexual complaints. The acupuncturist typically takes a comprehensive history and develops a complete history of your condition. An individualized plan of management is created and ongoing care often yields excellent results.

Traditional Chinese medicine specialists feel that sex drive and desire are from Yuan Chi. According to the book *Chi and Libido* by Tom Tam, Yuan Chi is defined as the genuine chi and can be thought of as the life essence provided at conception by both parents. Yuan Chi is housed in the kidney, and its primary function is to promote normative bodily growth and development as well as to maintain the health and vigor of all bodily functions. Yuan Chi can be diminished with time by a variety of different issues such as poor diet, excessive lifestyle, stress, and diseases such as cancer and their subsequent treatments.

When considering the complex issue of sexual function in women, treatment must be tailored to the specific patterns of imbalance that are revealed through tongue and pulse diagnosis as well as detailed history concerning diet, lifestyle, and medical and emotional health. Acupuncturists are specialized healthcare professionals who are required to complete 4 years of academic and clinical training before becoming eligible to take the rigorous state and licensing examinations. Strict standards are required to maintain their licenses. Needles, when used, are under strict healthcare regulations for maintaining sterile environments.

79. Can exercise be used to improve sexual function?

The obesity and overweight statistics of North American adults are alarming. Too many of us have gained more than a few pounds and we have developed into a nation of overweight couch potatoes. Of course, our bodies may have changed since our youth, but increased weight is clearly associated with a variety of health conditions: diabetes, hypertension, hypercholesterolemia, and heart disease.

Vigorous exercise can remarkably improve sexuality.

Besides the obvious health reasons, numerous recent studies have shown that regular, vigorous exercise can remarkably improve sexuality. Exercise has also been linked to decreased breast cancer rates. Exercise may enhance sexual performance and decrease sexual dysfunction from a physical, physiologic, and psychological perspective. A frequent and intense exercise program that focuses on cardiovascular and muscular endurance, muscular strength, and flexibility can allow for longer-lasting and more comfortable sex.

It is estimated that one sexual encounter actually burns approximately 150–200 calories, which is the amount of calories in two to three small chocolate chip cookies. Physical exercise improves physiologic sexual response and functioning by increasing circulation, which includes blood flow to the genital region. A recent study conducted by Cindy Meston at the University of Texas at Austin shows that when women have exercised vigorously for 20 minutes, they are more quickly aroused than when they have not exercised previously. Exercise has also been shown to reduce stress, improve self-esteem, and increase a personal sense of confidence. These positive psychological effects cause you to feel good about your personal, physical, and sexual attractiveness and ability.

Raye comments:

Regular exercise can not only do wonders for your mind and soul, but can definitely improve your complete sexual function. Exercise increases your blood flow, which will definitely help with circulation and performance. Another benefit to regular exercise is weight loss. And we all love that! It also makes a positive improvement on physical appearance, which will psychologically do wonders for your sexual function. I know it's hard to get motivated to go to the gym—I started with just walking, parking farther than my final destination. It was a gradual process to get to the gym. I just knew deep down inside that I needed to get my butt in the gym and work out, and I am happier now that I have committed to my health and know the benefits of exercise.

Using Tai Chi Chuan to Enhance Sexual Fitness

Sexual intimacy can be physically demanding; fatigue and tiredness can be reduced with regular exercise. Tai chi chuan has many benefits including increased flexibility, increased strength, and improved breathing. Tai chi chuan has also been linked to immune function, and increased relaxation, as well as encouraging whole body movements. Reduction of stress is also accomplished with tai chi chuan, resulting in peaceful serenity. Practicing tai chi chuan is also helpful in training your mind to be focused in the here-and-now, to be ever present in the moment and not wandering with your thoughts and interests. Staying focused during an intimate encounter is paramount. Movement, concentration, togetherness, and connectedness with your partner can be accomplished by practicing tai chi chuan. Try a class today with your significant other.

Too Much of Certain Types of Exercise May Be Hazardous to Your Sex Life

Recent emerging evidence, as presented and discussed by Dr. Irwin Goldstein, Director of Sexual Medicine at Alvarado

Hospital, suggests that excessive bike riding in women may actually be affecting their ability to perform sexually and achieve an orgasm. While the rider is placing her weight on the protruding nose of the bicycle seat, the pudendal nerve may become entrapped by pushing it consistently against the pubic bone. Some women who cycle long distances or do repetitive spinning classes report deep aching, burning, throbbing, numbness, or tingling in the pelvic area.

New types of bike seats are emerging; for example, saddle seats with gel saddles, cutouts, and padding are designed to relieve pressure on the perineum and other tender body parts.

PART EIGHT

Putting It All Together

My partner and I have different levels of sexual interest. How can we deal with sexual libido mismatch?

What are some general strategies to enhance intimacy and sexuality?

How can I promote lifelong sexual wellness and vitality?

More . . .

80. What is sexual boredom?

*Like most
activities,
sexual intimacy
can become
boring or stale
after a while.*

Like most activities, sexual intimacy can become boring or stale after a while. We often fall into what is often called a sexual rut, having sex in the same location, at the same time, and in the same position. Sex often becomes part of the plan; sometimes it is even scheduled on a regular basis even if the desire and interest are not present. Even if it is enjoyable, it can become boring and mundane, expected, with little excitement or variation.

In addition, some couples are paralyzed by sexual myths that have erroneously been perpetuated by society. Myths relating to culture—such as the belief that African American males are always well endowed and African American women are always interested in sexual play, or that French men and women are excellent lovers—influence how we view ourselves and our partners. Culture can also affect our communication and interactions.

Here are some practical suggestions that you can implement in your own sex life to help spice things up. Try changing locations if possible; have sex in the living room, in the shower or tub, or perhaps meet at a hotel for a quick sexual interlude. Experiment with different forms of stimulation: try massage or oral sex. Change your routine—how about a shower together? Read some erotic literature or watch a romantic movie. Try romance, seduction, or be adventurous with body paints and sexual games.

Try sex with the lights on. If you and your partner are typically night owls, try early morning sexual activity, which is often associated with improved arousal and performance as a result of heightened testosterone levels in the morning. Try fun exotic vacations like an African safari, rock climbing, or a stay at a romantic isolated beach.

Try a sexual date or quickie. Sexual quickies are planned sexual escapes that focus primarily on sexual interplay and arousal with orgasm. They can happen any place and at any time. Often, the surprise factor or fear of discovery can play a part in excitement. Clearly, there is a difference between quick sexual episodes and lengthy lovemaking sessions. The variety can complement and enhance the intimacy of the relationship. Lusty, fast encounters can also be satisfying for both partners. An excellent resource for some thoughtful ideas includes Tara Roth's book *Romance on the Run: Five Minutes of Quality Sex for Busy Couples.* Try something new and exciting today.

Raye comments:

Sexual boredom is when couples in relationships get in a rut. Just like everything in life, sex can become a routine—especially after being with your partner for a long period of time. I think people get almost too comfortable and instead of remembering what made your relationship have that fire initially, you let the fire go out. I think any relationship that is going to survive needs to have spice on both ends, and both partners need to communicate and constantly be willing to be adventurous, playful, and open to new ideas to keep the flame going. Men need to still be romantic. Don't forget it, and we as women shouldn't let them forget! It's about intimacy, courting, and sometimes the chase! They should keep doing the things that got us madly hooked on them in the first place. Don't men know how to be romantic any more or did that go out of style, too? And, no, snuggling on the couch watching boring football together is not romantic, sensual, or quality time! Don't forget about romance!

81. How can I improve my physical appearance to enhance sexual wellness?

The chubby hubby with a big belly may not be appealing, and the wife with an increased abdominal waist may not be as self-assured as she once was. Physical appearance is important to sexual attraction. We all can use a bit of fine-tuning and be sensitive to our partner's wants and likes. It is also important to understand that we all do change with time. The extra pounds not only change how we look but also can be contributors to chronic medical diseases such as heart problems and diabetes. Take a good hard look at yourself. Have you skipped the gym too often and had a few of those extra chocolate chip cookies? Are you carrying around a spare tire? Have you forgotten the number to the hair stylist?

Improving your physical appearance and attractiveness is not only for your partner but also for your self-esteem. Starting again with your exercise workouts, healthy diet, and self-grooming can do wonders for your self-esteem, not to mention your sex life. Both men and women have become interested and involved in the age of metrosexuality . Think about a renewed focus on your appearance where your hair is coiffed and combed, eyebrows are plucked or trimmed. Some have even gone as far as to preen pubic hair or trim underarm hair. It is not uncommon to see body hair removed or groomed. Waxing, shaving, and primping are not only for women—many men have jumped on the bandwagon and are attentive to their appearances as well. You do not need to go full force, but think about how you have let yourself go. How can you improve your personal appearance for your self–esteem?

82. My partner and I have different levels of sexual interest. How can we deal with sexual libido mismatch?

The quality of your relationship with your sexual partner is likely to have the biggest effect on your sexual libido and your frequency of intimacy.

When partners in a romantic relationship have different levels of desire or interest in sexual activities, it may be traceable to larger, more serious issues in the relationship. Communication is the key when you disagree in this area. Many experts agree that the quality of your relationship with your sexual partner is likely to have the biggest effect on your sexual libido and your frequency of intimacy.

If you're ready to try to get in sync with your partner about sexual desire and frequency and are trying to resolve some of your sexual health concerns, the first activity should be talking. Get to the basis of the sexual mismatch. Like many issues in relationships, communication and compromise are often the best solution and answer. Be careful and considerate in your approach. It is not only what you say but how you say it, and the method of discussion should be in a calm, nonaccusatory fashion. If your partner wants intimacy much more often than you do, try to come to some agreement so that neither partner is feeling pressured or neglected. Try to prevent any heightened emotional outbursts with undertones of anger, resentment, and distrust.

Focus on your own feelings and limitations without pointing the finger and being overly critical of your partner. Some practical suggestions to increase emotional connectedness are as follows:

- Increase your displays of affection: hug, kiss, caress, and compliment each other often.
- Reigniting passion may be awkward at first. Take your time, and focus on passion and intimacy rather than goals of intercourse or orgasm.
- Spending quality time together may help heighten your romantic connection.
- Share your sexual thoughts and desires as well as fantasies even if awkward at first. Listen without judgment.
- For the higher libido partner: try to accept no without personal offence and consider self-stimulation as an alternative acceptable sexual behavior and release.
- For the lower libido partner: consider engaging in some type of foreplay and sexual activity even if not 100% in the mood because some sexual research theory supports the notion that the more you engage in sex, the more likely you may desire it.

If you are still struggling and this is causing conflict in your relationship, do not be afraid to consult a sexual medicine specialist for mismatched libidos. Sometimes professional help with a counselor can also be beneficial.

Putting It All Together

May–December Relationships, Cradle Robbers, and Cougars Revised

May–December relationships often mean relationships in which there is a large age discrepancy between partners. Along with the cradle robber (older man with a young woman) and the cougar (older woman with young man), these types of relationships may sometimes lead to mismatch in libido. There is a considerable double standard in societal judgment regarding relationships in which there are huge age mismatches—society still frowns upon older women with younger boyfriends, whereas many congratulate older men with young girlfriends. Many assume that money, social status, or something else is behind the coupling; love and attraction are seldom mentioned in the backroom whispers.

Sometimes the age difference is not an issue, and couples with large age differences can navigate this difference when others, because of age, declining hormones, or superimposed medical, physical, and or psychological illnesses, succumb to mismatch in sexual desire and frequency. If there is any doubt as to the cause of the libido mismatch, do not hesitate to seek medical care and get a detailed sexual health evaluation and comprehensive treatment plan.

83. What are some general strategies to enhance intimacy and sexuality?

Some practical suggestions to optimize sexual functioning include limiting alcohol consumption, avoiding all tobacco, and delaying sexual activity until 2 or more hours after drinking alcohol or eating. See your healthcare provider and get a checkup to rule out underlying diseases that can affect your sexual response cycle. If you are taking medications, have them reassessed. If you take pain medications, perhaps try taking them 30 to 45 minutes before planned sexual activity. Keeping pain to a minimum is critical.

Some practical environmental changes that you can make is to preplan sexual activity. Intimacy should occur when your energy level is at its peak, fatigue is at a minimum, and your symptoms from chronic medical diseases are at their lowest. Often, intimate morning encounters are better because each partner may be well rested and sexual hormonal levels are at their highest. Take care to avoid the extremes of temperature. Try to experiment with pillows to ensure comfort while enjoying new, exciting sexual positions. You should not forget the importance of general health maintenance, so try a healthy, well-balanced diet, sleep well, and enjoy regular aerobic exercise.

The progression of intimacy is often seen as physical closeness (spending time together), emotional togetherness (sharing intimate thoughts and desires—what is your 5-year plan together as a couple?), sensual intimacy (nonthreatening sensual activities, such as erotic showers, **outercourse**, massage, and touching each other in pleasurable ways), and finally, sexual coupling or erotic sexual behavior with foreplay and intercourse. Try starting by spending time together and make spending time as a couple a priority; take a walk, have a date, or organize your hectic calendars so that you have special time together that is focused on your partnership. Put financial concerns, mortgage, and work issues on the back burner and focus on what brought you together and what your future goals will be. Plan romantic getaways, fantasize about the future. Be spontaneous. Try to be together even when apart: brief calls, love notes in lunch bags, or computer chats can help closeness even when travel separates you as a couple.

Next plan some sensual activities. An erotic shower or massage may be exciting and an activity that you have not done together in many years. Slowly progress to sexual play and do not forget foreplay and other sexual activities.

Outercourse

Sexual activities other than intercourse; fondling, touching, kissing, oral and genital play are often considered outercourse. It can be promoted as a means of sexual activity that prevents unwanted pregnancy and that can minimize sexually transmitted diseases.

Communication in and outside of the bedroom is important to help keep a relationship and marriage alive and well.

A word about communication: communication in and outside of the bedroom is important to help keep a relationship and marriage alive and well. Some practical suggestions include these: don't argue in front of the children, think and filter your words before you speak, take some time to cool down, and make a date to chat about problems or concerns. It is important to always listen and focus, and it may be helpful to pick a time when communication will happen uninterrupted when everyone is level headed. Also, do not forget to compliment each other! Appreciate each other on a daily basis.

84. What are some thoughts about condoms?

An article in the lay journal *The Female Patient* titled "Modern Male Condoms: Not Your Father's Rubbers" is an excellent summary of new and exciting ideas concerning condoms and their use. This article details the eye-catching advertising and racy packaging that make the use of condoms more appealing and addresses many issues and complaints that consumers have. The authors also address the fact that now is the time to make condoms fashionable, both for pregnancy prevention and sexually transmitted disease prevention.

Some women may be allergic to latex or be latex sensitive and may experience itchiness or other distressing symptoms after intercourse with a condom. They may also get frequent yeast infections and be prone to other vaginal infections. For these special women, polyurethane condoms are the best choice. Also, a special lubricant with no additives can be the best option. In clinical trials, the polyurethane condom provided pregnancy protection equal to that of the latex condom but had breakage and spillage rates that were significantly higher. It is also important to remember that antifungal therapies, all vaginal antibiotic treatments that are placed intravaginally, and estrogen creams that are petroleum based may affect the integrity of condoms.

Condoms come in all shapes, colors, and sizes, and about 5% of the users in the United States complain of constriction with standard-sized condoms. For these men, newer sizes are available including magnum and extra large. Condoms now have new flavors for oral sex; strawberry and cherry are often the favorites. All colors of the rainbow are now available for sexual visual excitement and have a wide variety of lubricants and moisturizers within their packaging. Trojan has also come out with a new exciting line and offers a wide variety of selections.

There is no better time to use condoms, both for sexual pleasure and fulfillment and also to prevent pregnancy and sexually transmitted diseases. For more information about condoms consult www.condomania.com or www.condomdepot.com.

Raye comments:

Condoms are talked about a lot more now than ever before. They are everywhere from magazine advertisements, commercials, bathrooms, to nurses handing them out at schools. Safe sex is being promoted and condoms are being distributed like they are a piece of gum. They come in all different shapes, sizes, colors, and textures now. Most men, even though they know they should wear one, still make excuses and hate them.

85. What are some sexual accessories?

There are many sexual accessories available for sexual enhancement, some designed for her and some for him. Self-stimulators are discussed in depth elsewhere, and there are many other products available. Nipple and G-spot stimulators are popular for many women. For men, the products range from steel constricting rings, which are placed around the base of the penis to decrease blood flow and promote erections, to anal stimulators, which can enhance the male G-spot stimulation.

Putting It All Together

Some other suggestions for couple activities include role-play, secret dates, and the use of costumes, or even masks, feathers, or ticklers. Sexual fantasies with costumes, set design, and other role-playing techniques are often used by couples exploring this facet of sexual play. Chocolate body paint or honey dust by Kama Sutra are also exciting activities for couples; take turns painting each other, and then savor the flavors. The chocolate comes with a brush and three flavors of chocolate—light, dark, and white—and can be painted on the body in creative patterns, and then can be eaten off. Honey dust is used with a feather duster so that you can sprinkle and dust your partner with pure honey powder.

Sexual games come in all shapes and sizes.

Sexual games come in all shapes and sizes, and a variety of games can be purchased at your local sexual accessory store or on the Internet. Some interesting ones include card games, sexually explicit dice, and other racy sex card games to heat up your intimate evenings. Sexual dominos, aromatic bath scents, and bath salts can also be used. Clever card games and coupons can also be exchanged between couples to help enhance the sexual atmosphere. For the inexperienced, try sensual aromatic massage lotions or other bath products.

86. What is oral sex?

Fellatio

Latin word for the sexual act between the mouth of one person and the penis of another.

Cunnilingus

Sexual contact between the tongue or mouth of one person and the vulva/clitoral tissue of another.

According to the Revolution Health informational publication, *oral sex* can be defined as the sexual act of placing your mouth on your partner's genitals or stimulating an erotic zone with one's mouth. **Fellatio** is the term used to describe oral sex performed on a male, whereas **cunnilingus** is oral sex performed on a woman. There are a variety of ways to perform oral sex on your partner. Couples can individually arouse each other's genitals one at a time, or they can do it at the same time. Many couples enjoy this kind of pleasurable sexual interaction. For some, this is the only form of sexual pleasure.

Many couples have preconceived notions about oral sex; some think it is erotic whereas others believe it is a dirty act. Discuss your interest or lack thereof concerning oral stimulation with your partner in an open, comfortable, nonsexual scenario. What you do like about his or her technique, how can it be improved to suit your personal erotic needs? Whether you talk about oral sex with your partner before, during, or after the act, above all, bear in mind that you should always be gentle, thoughtful, and sensitive in your feedback.

How to Give Pleasure to a Man

When it comes to arousing your male partner, each man enjoys different activities. Some enjoy kissing, caressing, sucking, massaging, or licking the penis, shaft, or the glans (head) of the penis. For many men, the scrotum is also an extremely erotic and sensual zone, and gentle stroking or massaging of this area can be pleasing. Change and alter rhythm. Discuss with your partner what he enjoys and experiment with different techniques. Some men enjoy stimulation of the perineum or the area between the base of the scrotum and the anus. Gentle tickling touch may be arousing to some men, while others find this unexciting. Women should have control of the depth and extent of oral penetration to minimize fear of gagging.

How to Give Pleasure to a Woman

Like men, no two women are the same when it comes to oral stimulation; what feels exciting to one may be annoying to another. Many enjoy pressure or light touch with the tongue to the clitoral area, whereas others prefer a more deep and rapid touch. Some men do not even know where the clitoris is, so women may need to educate their partners as to what feels exciting, sensual, and arousing while gently informing them about which techniques are displeasing.

A Word About Safety

Oral sex does pose a disease risk. Although the risks are low, many healthcare professionals cannot exactly quantify the risk. The Centers for Disease Control and Prevention (CDC) states that the risk of transmitting human immunodeficiency virus (HIV) through performing or receiving oral sex is less than that of unprotected anal or vaginal sex. They do reiterate that HIV and other sexually transmitted disease (STD) transmission (including human papillomavirus [HPV], herpes, gonorrhea, syphilis, and Chlamydia infection) can occur. You should be careful if you or your partner have any active outbreaks on your mouth, lips, or genitals, such as sores, warts, ulcers, or weeping lesions.

The CDC recommends that if people do have oral sex, partners use latex condoms (on male partners) or latex barriers such as a latex sheet, dental dam, or cut-open condom to cover the female's parts. This may not, in fact, be desirable or feasible for couples in committed, stable, monogamous relationships. You and your partner know each other, develop sexual communication and trust, and keep the dialogue ongoing. Some in new relationships even advocate testing for sexually transmitted diseases.

It's always important to remember that oral sex on pregnant women should be avoided in the last trimester and partners should take care never to blow air into the vagina. Doing so could cause a serious medical complication called an air embolism, which may threaten the health of the woman or the baby.

87. What are some sexual positions?

Most couples have a sexual routine or script that they are used to. Coming home with flowers or chocolate signals what will follow: romantic dinner, some brief foreplay, and then penetration and ejaculation mostly in the same position at the same time of day, and maybe even the same day of each week. Many couples have become accustomed to using only one sexual position.

Varying sexual positioning can be very helpful to spice up a boring or ho-hum sexual relationship.

Varying sexual positioning can be very helpful to spice up a boring or ho-hum sexual relationship. Most couples have intercourse in the missionary position (man on top of the woman), which was promoted by the missionaries for procreation not recreation. This position facilitates deep penetration so as to deposit sperm near the cervix to facilitate fertilization; many women do not find this position enjoyable because neither the clitoral nor the vaginal G-spot is stimulated. It also limits female mobility and her control, and it may also affect the quality of thrusting on the man's part. A modification of this position is the seated missionary as well as knee-to-chest position.

Face-to-face is another excellent position that can enhance communication, touch, and speech. Female superior, or when the women is on top of the man, who is on his back, is also an excellent position because it enables men to have free hands to stimulate the clitoral and breast tissues. Men who have issues with premature ejaculation and those who ejaculate quickly may also benefit from this position because it can increase the man's ability to maintain an erection and prolong the feelings of ejaculation. Many women find this position enjoyable and empowering because they can control the force and depth of penetration. Standing, sexual entry from behind, or spooning are also other sexual positions that you can explore and enjoy.

Of course, there is a wide variety of variations, and sexual exploration is the key. Some positioning books that are excellent resources include *The Joy of Sex* and *The Multiorgasmic Couple*.

88. What are some anal sex issues and answers?

Even in a time of increasing sexual acceptance and open discussion, anal sex remains clouded in mystery with a lot of misconception for both receptive and active partners. According to the National Center for Health Statistics, 34% of American men and 30% of women aged 15 to 44 report having had anal sex at least once. Many women enjoy this sexual activity as their primary sexual activity. The myths that no one is performing anal intercourse and that anal sex is "gay sex" are clearly incorrect.

Anal sex can be extremely pleasurable.

Anal sex can be extremely pleasurable. The anus contains an abundant nerve supply and is an erogenous zone in both men and women. Anal sex should never be painful, and it requires preparation, patience, and skill, according to Susan Kellogg Spadt, director of Sexual Medicine at the Pelvic and Sexual Health Institute of Philadelphia. The walls of the anus are not as pliable as the vaginal walls and neither does the anus produce its own lubrication like the vaginal tissues.

Unprotected anal sex is considered an extremely high risk sexual behavior and can be associated with increased transmission of many sexually transmitted diseases. The anal canal also contains bacteria that can cause urinary tract and prostate infections in men who don't use condoms. Women should never place anything from the anus into the vagina without washing, and condoms should never be reused.

To stay safe and enjoy anal pleasure, be sure to use a well-lubricated latex condom every time. Never reuse any condoms. If you have vaginal or oral intercourse after anal sex, use a new condom. You should never have unprotected anal sex, even if you and your partner are in a committed exclusive relationship and are disease-free. Use a barrier, such as a dental dam, natural rubber latex sheet, cut-open condom, or even plastic wrap if you are engaging in oral–anal sexual activities. Be certain to cleanse sex toys with soap and water before placing them in the anus. The anal sphincters are tight bands of muscle, and trying to penetrate them in a hurry or roughly can lead to pain and tearing, so relaxation with deep rhythmic breathing is essential. Slow down and communicate. Use lubrication often.

Many people like to shower before anal sex, and some use enemas to further clean the anus and rectum. Have a towel handy for easy cleanup. Avoid using alcohol or drugs or other substances during anal sexual activity, which may impair good judgment and affect communication.

Sexual accessories can sometimes become lost or lodged in the anal canal and can become a medical emergency. Always ensure that toys do have a base and can be easily removed. Never place foreign objects in the vagina or anal canal. If you experience severe pain or bleeding, see a healthcare professional and get an evaluation and necessary treatment.

Sometimes one partner wants to engage in anal sex and the other partner feels uncomfortable about this activity. There is no clear answer how to handle this issue, but you should communicate and share your feelings openly and honestly with your partner. According to Dr. Kellogg, you can and should begin with experimentation by touching or massaging the anal opening without penetration; this can be extremely erotic experience.

89. What are polyamorous relationships?

Polyamorous relationships are making a new resurgence in the public! They are gaining attention and sometimes criticism from the lay public and politicians, who rarely know much about their situations and relationships. Polyamorous relationships are relationships in which people engage in openly nonmonogamous relationships with partners. They have also been called "expanded relationships." Some live together, others do not; some share homes and financial responsibilities, whereas others do not; childrearing may also be shared in some situations. The couples tend to have modified sexual boundaries and engage in satisfying sexual relationships with different partners.

Some typical characteristics of the polyamorous person include white, upper to middle class, professionally educated, liberal views, and often engaged in computer-related fields of work or study. Some of the women are bisexual and the men may be bisexual. Ideally, polyamorous relationships are conducted with open awareness and emotional attachments to multiple people.

Polyamorous relationships, in which both men and women can enjoy multiple intimate, loving, and caring relationships that are sexually satisfying, may be deemed more intimate and emotionally connected than the other concept known as "swinging." The number of people who are involved in poly relationships varies and can be two, three, four, or more. The more people that are involved, the more complex the sexual and living situation becomes. Also, with more people involved the relationship is more likely to become unstable. The most common form is the "open relationship" where the couple usually cohabitate and have outside relationships with other people. Triads are perpetual three-ways commonly known as a *ménage a trois*; quads often form when two couples join together. Quads tend to be unstable and often end in relationship termination.

Other unconventional arrangements in marriages are common and can include "managed monogamy." Some couples may enjoy above-the-waist rules (touching another above the waist line is permissible), don't-ask-don't-tell policies (people in committed relationships may have discrete outside relationships but do not inform their partners), and 50-mile rules (partners cannot engage in outside sexual encounters with anyone within a 50-mile radius of the couple's home town).

Swinging was popular in the 1970s and is when couples engage in partner swapping with other people or couples. A trinogamous relationship is one in which three people have committed to be monogamous with each other. Other couples engage in bringing other partners into their marital bed, and others allow for extramarital affairs with partner consent.

No matter what your arrangement, honesty and communication are key, as is protection from sexually transmitted diseases. These arrangements are not for everyone and may often lead to increased conflict or marital discord.

90. Should we enter into the sexual fringe?

Entering the fringe, or engaging in what is considered outside normative or conservative sexual practices, may be of interest to you and your partner. It is best to discuss your interests and desires and to formulate a mutually respected and agreed-upon plan of action.

Bondage and leather activities are sometimes considered out of the realm of normative acceptable sexual practices. Normative practices are often defined by the culture to which you ascribe. Increased marital discomfort can occur when one party is ready to enter the fringe and the other is scared, apprehensive, or not interested. Discuss and communicate openly. Honesty about fantasy and sexual exploration is essential.

One way to communicate about entering the sexual fringe is to explore erotic material together as a couple. To spice up a somewhat dull sex life, some try exploring together—a trip to the local video store may be all that you need to spice up and sexually charge your evenings of boredom and ho-hum sex. Most videos can be rented without embarrassment. Some women do not find these types of videos enjoyable and they can affect self-esteem if their partner admires and is excited by the ideal movie starlet. Other couples try magazines, films, or books, and the act of sharing these together may be enlightening.

If you are too concerned about the corner store video arcade, try the Internet or mail order. Some sexually exciting movies include *9½ Weeks*; *10*; *American Gigolo*; *Sex, Lies and Videotape*; *Striptease*; and *Wild Things*. Other soft- or hard-core erotic adult entertainment may also be available and can be viewed together.

Honesty about fantasy and sexual exploration is essential.

Putting It All Together

Erotic Sexy Striptease Pole Dancing

There is a new exercise plan available: sexy pole-dancing classes and the Striptease Workout. Basically, these types of aerobic classes involve intense exercise and incorporate pole dancing and sexy moves into the routine. During these erotic dances, women gain confidence in their sexuality and sensuality in a comfortable, nonthreatening environment. The inner burlesque is released and eye contact, body language, hip movements, and posing are encouraged.

Typically, different types of dance are also included such as belly dancing, cabaret, and yoga. Women of all shapes, sizes, and backgrounds can enjoy these activities and most do not have a stripper's body. Partners are rather excited when their wives or girlfriends return home, and many are surprised by the interesting results. Check out www.sfactor.com and www.dgentertainment.ca. The program allows women to explore sexuality with a sense of humor, and the results of improved sexual intimacy are remarkable.

Some other areas of exploration that can help reduce sexual boredom or expand a sexual repertoire include erotic bars/night clubs, strip or sex clubs, erotic theaters, body modification/tattooing, visiting a museum of sex, sexual art, dominance and submission role playing, and Russian and Turkish baths. Use your imagination and let your inner sexual desires come to the surface. Discuss and communicate with your partner and explore in a safe, comfortable environment.

91. What about pornography, videos, and magazines—are they friends or foes?

Pornography has different meanings for the sexes.

Pornography has different meanings for the sexes; reactions can be different as are sexual desires. For women, it may be degrading and demeaning showing women in compromising situations and may even affect their self-esteem by reinforcing feeling of inability to live up to the perfect depiction of the idealized women with perfect breasts and voluptuous body.

For men, it maybe an enhancement, an escape to fantasy without any further significance in sexual interest.

Porn gazing can become an issue with couples and can affect relationship intimacy and connectedness. For conflicted couples, pornography can be destructive, yet for some, erotica can be shared and can enhance sexual dynamics and repertoires between partners. Erotica, pornographic pictures, websites, and other fantasy material either in cyberspace or in print are readily available both on the Internet and at your local corner store. According to comScore, 66% of Internet-using men between the ages of 18 and 34 years look at online porn at least once a month. In a 2003 issue of *Journal of Sex and Marital Therapy*, Bridges and associates found that although most women weren't bothered by their partner's X-rated interests, a small few were extremely distressed by it. According to *Psychology Today*, a common response women may feel is a strong sense of violation including feelings of betrayal.

Men may explain pornography as an exploration of fantasy and curiosity. For men, looking at naked women may be done partly out of boredom, as a replacement or stimulus for self-stimulation, or as a substitute for infrequent sexual activity. According to David Schnarch, author of *Resurrecting Sex and the Passionate Marriage*, pornography can enhance or promote emotional and sexual intimacy. Schnarch says that couples can develop a deeper sexual connection with the use of erotic images. Erotica, and the couple's sensual fantasies, are used to help them grow, intensify their sexual relationship, and improve the dynamic between them. Fantasy is an important facet of the healthy sex life, and pornography can help create or inspire sexual scenarios and modify sexual scripts that have become stale and boring.

With the ease and privacy of the Internet, many women are now active participants in using erotica and pornography. There is little research on how men feel about their female partner's porn use. According to Pamela Paul in her book

Putting It All Together

Pornified: How Pornography Is Transforming Our Lives, Our Relationships, and Our Families, many men hope their partners approve or tolerate their own use of porn but may be critical of a girlfriend or wife who uses pornography herself. Some men may get more aroused with their partners' active use of erotica whereas others are concerned by its implications in the relationship. In a 2004 *Elle*–MSNBC.com poll, 6 in 10 men were concerned about their partner's interest in Internet pornography.

Some individuals are vulnerable to compulsive sexual behavior, and abuse of Internet pornography sites is not uncommon. Online pornography can become an obsession. Best advice is to examine what pornography means to the dynamic of your relationship, and to you personally. Why is there anger? Is the sexual repertoire scripted and boring? Predictable? Ask yourself whether you need more experimentation. Passion? Are you restless and discontent? What can you as a couple do about it? Open the lines of communication and begin a frank discussion. Pornography is not all bad or detrimental to the relationship. Pornography and erotica can be helpful in spicing up a boring or mundane, dry sex life. Exploration of your sexual fantasies can be a useful treatment tool to help nurture aspects of your sexual relationship.

92. How do I set the stage for sexuality?

Creating a sensual environment can be accomplished in a variety of ways. Understanding your own personal needs and wants as well as the interests of your partner is helpful.

Feng shui is the ancient Chinese practice believed to utilize the laws of both heaven (astronomy) and earth (geography) to help you improve your life by receiving positive energy. The modern practice of feng shui is the art of arranging objects (such as furniture) to help people achieve personal goals though a harmonious environment. Feng shui knowledge can be used to create a nice, aesthetically pleasing environment; this allows for a sense of balance and warmth and makes certain that furniture matches the room size.

Most people have intercourse in the bedroom, so some important items to remember to include are as follows:

- A large, high-quality mattress is essential. Ensure that is comfortable for you and your partner. It should not be too hard or too soft.
- Mood lighting (dimmers should be on master bedroom lighting) and cotton or silky sheets are also must-haves for a sensual environment.
- Artwork that is serene and depicting loving romantic scenes should also be placed in the bedroom.
- Personal symbols of love, happiness, wedding, or honeymoon pictures, for example, should fill the room with serenity and loving compassion.

Some things to avoid, according to feng shui principles, that may affect sexual intimacy include a storage room aligned with the master bedroom (this will decrease energy and may lead to depression or money loss), toilet facing your bed, lots of storage underneath the bed, irregular-shaped rooms with many angles and missing corners, or dead or dried flowers. All these factors create negative energy and may affect libido and sexual function.

You also do not want a noisy environment, or one that is ruined by much noise and air pollution (disruption of sleep and mood). Air quality should be good, and your bed should not be aligned with a window because the lack of privacy may hinder sexual intimacy. A healthy, healing environment can create a place that will promote kissing, touching, and intercourse. An environment can create a balance of energy and promote sexual wellness.

Putting It All Together

Aromatherapy can be used as an adjunct to enhance the mood: try a few drops of your favorite essential oil in a water-filled spray bottle and scent the room. A few drops on your pillow or on a light bulb ring can provide a sensual aroma to a boring or dull room. Scent your lingerie or prepare your own signature massage oil. Some of the preferred oils to promote sensuality and seduction include clary sage, jasmine, rose, sandalwood, ylang-ylang, and cinnamon. Scented massage oils or lotions also can be incorporated into the sexual repertoire.

Romantic music may also set the stage for a perfect sexual encounter. Sometimes couples have a special song or one that has special lyrics that can be played to enhance the mood. Old wonderful memories can resurface. Some artists of love songs include Andréa Bocelli, Michael Buble, Celine Dion, Barbara Streisand, Frank Sinatra, and Enya. Candles, aromatic and scented massage oils, and sexy lingerie for both him and her can also help seal the mood of romance and love.

93. How can color therapy be useful for sexuality?

According to About.com, color therapy, also known as chromotherapy, is classified as a vibrational healing technique that incorporates the use of energies within living organisms such as plants, gemstones and crystals, water, sunlight, and sound. Color is simply a form of visible light. The color of our clothes and our environment can influence how we feel and how we act. Sexuality is no exception. A therapist who is specifically trained in color therapy applies light and color to balance energy in the areas of our bodies that are lacking vibrance, be it physical, emotional, spiritual, or mental.

Color therapy is the practice by which colors that you wear or those in your environment promote feelings within each individual. Think about the colors you wear and the mood you are in. Do they complement each other? What about the décor in your bed chamber? Is it calming and soothing and colored as a place designed for love, sensuality, and nurturance? Do you feel sexy in this room? According to the Chakra Color website, several colors have meaning when it comes to enhancement of sexuality:

- Blue is cooling to body and mind and promotes relaxation. It is often used in the interior of the home and bedroom because it enhances the quiet mind.
- Purple is associated with self-esteem and spirituality.
- Green is the color of nature and is associated with tranquility and balance. It is a relaxing color for the brain, a healing color, because it soothes the body, mind, and spirit.
- Orange represents happiness, passion, and extroversion. Orange can stimulate creativity, vitality, and also male and female sensuality. Some experts feel that visualizing orange can eliminate depression and can bring joy and happiness.
- Yellow is associated with creativity and optimism and may enhance mood. Yellow is empowering and the symbol of the sun.
- Pink is the color of sensuality.
- Red is thought to be a powerful color of physical nature and is energizing and can be associated with deep emotions like love and anger. Red is often viewed as the symbol of life and courage, passion, and love.

Gemstones and Sexuality

Smoky quartz, the color of which ranges from light to dark shades of brown and gray, is often attributed the ability to neutralize negativity and also activates survival instincts. Some gemologists believe that the smoky crystals ground light force, transmitting energy into the physical body, enhancing focusing and concentration. They may eliminate fatigue and diminish procrastination. Some gemologists believe that smoky crystals can increase sexuality and fertility. Think about getting a small piece of smoky quartz today for your bedroom.

Putting It All Together

Diamonds are considered the modern symbol of eternal love. Carnelian gemstones are associated with increased sexual libido. Yellow zircon is thought to attract love into your life. Garnet, rhodonite, rose quartz, and clear quartz crystals have also been associated with enhanced love, passion, and human connectedness.

94. . . . It's not sex. . . it's intimacy. How do you focus on pleasure rather than performance?

As discussed earlier in the book, the goals of sexual wellness are to increase human connectedness and relationship togetherness rather than sexual intercourse. For some, sex may not be critical whereas for others the lack of communication may be troublesome. One of the critical issues you should focus on is sexual communication; discuss openly and honestly with your partner about getting what you want and need. Listen and communicate with your partner. Add spice and adventure—not criticism.

Many couples focus on goals such as orgasm, and their sexual script becomes preset and on automatic pilot. It's a routine that becomes boring after many years. Sex becomes a chore. The *escalator of sexual performance* is a term I use to discuss how one activity leads to the next, almost without thought or consideration. Bring home chocolates or flowers, have a nice meal, shower, kiss and hug in bed after a few minutes of your favorite television show. Next comes lights out with minimal foreplay; intercourse is rushed in the same position, and the whole sexual interlude culminates in orgasm about 5 to 10 minutes after it began. It's predictable, boring, often mechanical, and not pleasurable.

Rather than get on with another orgasm, you can focus on the concept of the wheel of pleasure. Like a wheel that rotates constantly, there are many places to get on and off. Spice it up, focus on sexual unpredictability. Have oral sex, outercourse. Maybe spend hours in romantic embrace without orgasm.

Focus on pleasure rather than performance. Focus on outercourse not intercourse.

Do not forget the power of the healing touch. It is known from medical research that the human brain releases natural endorphins in a surge following orgasm, meditation, and exercise. Men tend to release endorphins 20 to 30 seconds after orgasm, whereas women release endorphins up to 20 minutes after orgasm. Humans need connectedness, intimacy, and a sense of closeness. Focus on sensual touch. Deprivation of touch in men leads to aggressive behavior, whereas women who do not experience loving touch may become sad and depressed. Keeping stress to a minimum is also important. Use all your senses, touch and focus on pleasure rather than performance.

Focus on pleasure rather than performance.

95. How do we make sex a priority and make time for sex important?

What is time management? Everyone is limited by time. We all have an enormously long list that we never seem to be able to get accomplished. Work, family, social, and business commitments all accumulate, and then add those activities to the usual activities of daily living, and we are pressed for time. Do not forget the laundry, cooking, cleaning, and homework checking. We all have 60 seconds in a minute, 60 minutes in an hour, 24 hours in a day, and 168 hours in a week to get all that we do done. When we do not have enough time in the day, we stop having sex and sleep less—both activities that we need in times of stress.

Sex is important in your overall quality of life. Here are a few practical suggestions to help you manage your calendar and make yourself and sex a priority. Scheduled intimate time or planned intimacy is often better than no intimacy at all. Breaking your script and having sex at different times can also be spontaneous and exciting.

Putting It All Together

- Manage yourself and your choices. Set priorities and learn to say no to commitments both socially and professionally.
- Get a calendar and write it down.
- Begin by setting realistic goals; do not create impossible situations. Do not overschedule.
- Make a to-do list. Set reminders and avoid noisy environments.
- Avoid distractions, focus, and minimize possible interruptions—turn off your phone and the television.
- If you are feeling overwhelmed, reassess the number and types of projects you are involved in. Streamline.
- Minimize bodily stress. Become an active exerciser and improve your physical fitness.
- Meet your lover at home for some lunchtime loving.

Sometimes you may feel out of your comfort zone. Initially, it may feel abnormal for you to leave the sink filled with dirty dishes; but feeling connected with your partner or feeling the caress of your partner is often more important. Chores and other obligations should wait until another time. Make sex an important part of your routine. Making time for intimacy and passionate love will enhance your overall quality of life and sense of well-being. You will be surprised how it can help your overall efficiency.

Making time for intimacy and passionate love will enhance your overall quality of life and sense of well-being.

96. How do I relax and reduce fatigue so that I am receptive to sexual activity?

Sleep and fatigue are often major contributors to decreased sexual interest and desire. People rarely sleep properly, and new data support the notion that too little or too much sleep can be linked to the development of medical illnesses or even premature death. Poor sleep leads to daytime anxiety, restlessness, and irritability, all of which can affect your relationship. It is critical to pay special attention to good sleep behaviors and try to maintain good sleep techniques. Here are some helpful strategies:

- Go to bed and get up at the same time each day.
- Get regular exercise each day in the morning. There is good evidence that regular exercise improves restful sleep. This includes stretching and aerobic exercise.
- Get regular exposure to outdoor or bright light, especially in the late afternoon.
- Keep the temperature in your bedroom cool; keep it quiet, dark, and comfortable.
- Use your bed only for sleep and sex.
- Use a relaxation exercise like muscle relaxation, warm soaks, or imagery just before going to sleep.
- Avoid competitive games, watching television, or action adventure movies before going to bed.
- Leave important discussions with a loved one for the morning or afternoon.
- Avoid caffeine. It hides in many sources such as coffee, tea, and chocolate. Do not use alcohol as a sleep aid.
- Do not take another person's sleeping pills, and avoid daytime naps. Do not take over-the-counter sleeping pills without your doctor's knowledge.

Snoring can often be the reason why couples do not share a bed together. The noise may be unbearable and force loving couples into separate bedrooms. Snoring may be the prime issue that takes away from restful slumber, and it may be an indicator of some underlying medical concern. Both men and women who suffer from chronic heavy snoring should seek medical attention from a sleep center and have a comprehensive workup to rule out more serious conditions such as sleep apnea or a deviated septum.

97. Do I need a sexual consultation with a specialist?

You may wonder when it is time to seek professional help with sexual concerns. Sometimes you may have attempted to improve your sexual desire or lessen the pain you have experienced with intercourse, but the problems persist or worsen. Other times, the symptoms are severe or troublesome and your concern should be addressed. Vaginal bleeding or medication-induced sexual dysfunction should signal the time to consult a sexual healthcare professional. Referral for an evaluation by a subspecialist may be appropriate for certain clinical conditions.

Consultants can include oncologists, social services providers, nutritionists, exercise therapists, and psychiatrists. A list of clinicians and ancillary staff who are sensitive to sexual issues should be readily available for patients who take part in sexual rehabilitation programs. Providers need to reassure patients and their partners that even at the end of life when intercourse may not be feasible, intimacy and emotional closeness should be encouraged. Sexual complaints are often complex and often require the joint treatment effort from a medical professional and a psychotherapist who are trained in the field of sexual medicine.

98. Where can I seek help for myself and my partner?

Choosing the correct healthcare professional for your specific complaint takes careful consideration.

Many healthcare providers claim to be sexual experts, so choosing the correct healthcare professional for your specific complaint takes careful consideration. Medical doctors such as gynecologists and urologists sometimes have a special interest in sexual medicine. Mental healthcare professionals such as psychologists, social workers, and psychiatrists can also be helpful in treating sexual problems.

Be certain to verify credentials because qualifications and categories often change from state to state and location to location. The doctors who have chosen to specialize in sexual medicine often are compassionate and empathic. Sex therapists are mental healthcare providers who have specialized training in the diagnosis and treatment of sexual complaints.

Contact the American Association of Sex Educators, Therapists and Counselors (AASECT, www.aasect.org) and the Society for Sex Therapy and Research (SSTAR, www.sstarnet.org) for trained therapists in your neighborhood. Check the credentials of the specialist you plan to see and verify whether they take insurance.

Perhaps most important, do not be afraid to seek medical professional help. There are highly skilled sexual healthcare experts who understand that intimacy and connectedness are paramount to quality of life. Have the courage to seek help and restore your sexuality and sensuality.

99. How can I promote lifelong sexual wellness and vitality?

Lifelong sexual wellness is a commitment to yourself, your partner, and your relationship. Boredom is always a threat. Try to keep doing new and exciting things with your partner—not only does this increase hormones and neurotransmitters that can enhance intimacy and your relationship, but it can lead to decreased sexual boredom. Novelty triggers the transmitter dopamine to be released from the brain, which can stimulate feelings of connectedness and attraction and can enhance bonding. Ride a rollercoaster, dance naked in the living room, and use your imagination. Novel experiences shared together as a committed couple can increase closeness and increase sensual and sexual feelings.

You know the drill: eat all the right foods and get a lot of aerobic exercise and you'll live to a ripe old age. But apparently, there's more to good health than physical activity and good nutrition. Here are a few ways to boost your health and your long-term sexual satisfaction:

- Maintain social and community ties. Numerous studies have linked social support to improved immune function, longevity, a lower risk of heart disease, and speedier recovery from serious illness and surgery. In fact, a 1999 study in the *British Medical Journal* found that socially active individuals were just as healthy as their

Putting It All Together

counterparts who exercised regularly, and that social engagement was more important than blood pressure and cholesterol levels in determining longevity. These connections should be genuine: casual acquaintances and cocktail party chatter are no substitutes for fast friends and abiding relationships.

- Get a pet. The Centers for Disease Control and Prevention reports that having a pet can lower your blood pressure, decrease levels of cholesterol and triglycerides, and moderate feelings of loneliness. A 1999 study at the University of Buffalo showed that cats and dogs reduced blood pressure and heart rate in a group of high-stress stockbrokers.

- Take a vacation. A study published in 2005 in the *Wisconsin Medical Journal* found that women who took a vacation only once in 2 years had a higher risk of depression and stress than those who took two or more vacations a year. They were more likely to report lower marital satisfaction as well. And vacations are good for the heart—both for men and women. Women who take two or more vacations a year have half the risk of developing coronary heart disease or other serious heart problems.

- Laugh out loud. In *Anatomy of an Illness*, famed magazine editor Norman Cousins wrote that 10 minutes of belly laughter bought him 2 hours of pain-free sleep. Research at Loma Linda University in California has shown that laughter increases the number and activity level of the body's natural killer cells and reduces stress hormones that have been linked to heart disease.

- Pray or meditate. Although scientific proof of the efficacy of prayer lags behind claims, a 2001 study in the *British Medical Journal* reports that saying the rosary (or repeating yoga mantras) may be good for the heart by synchronizing breathing with cardiovascular rhythms. Proponents of the health benefits of prayer say it improves coping mechanisms and produces better health outcomes. Numerous studies have reported multiple health benefits from meditation (particularly Transcendental Meditation), among them stress reduction, improved recovery from surgery, lower blood pressure, improved pain management, and a longer lifespan.

- Get married or find a lifetime companion. Marriage and long-term relationships have been shown to reduce illnesses and increase longevity. People with healthy sex lives also have increased longevity and decreased depression rates.

100. Where can I go to learn more about the issues discussed in this book?

The resources listed here are what I recommend to my patients during the course of their treatment. Accessing them can provide you with a foundation of organizations, information, and sources that I hope will help you in your quest for sexual wellness and vitality. Enjoy the lifelong journey.

Some Important Websites

Southern California Center for Sexual Health and Survivorship Medicine: www.thesexualhealthcenter.com (949) 764-9300

> Dr. Krychman accepts all major health insurances and sees patients from all over California, the United States, and the world. Please call to schedule an appointment or to address your concerns.

Alexander Foundation: www.thealexanderfoundation.com

American Association for Marriage and Family Therapy: www.aamft.org

American Association of Sex Educators, Counselors and Therapists: www.aasect.org

American Cancer Society: www.cancer.org

People with healthy sex lives also have increased longevity and decreased depression rates.

Putting It All Together

American College of Obstetrics and Gynecology: www.acog.org

American Society for Reproductive Medicine: www.asrm.org

Black Women's Health Imperative: www.blackwomenshealth.org

Condomania: www.condomania.com

Contraception Online: www.contraceptiononline.org

Female Sexual Dysfunction Online: www.femalesexualdysfunctiononline.org

Gay and Lesbian Medical Association: www.glma.org

Good Vibrations: www.goodvibes.com

International Academy of Sex Research: www.iasr.org

International Society for the Study of Women's Sexual Health: www.isswsh.org

Kinsey Institute: www.kinseyinstitute.org

Lesbian Health Research Center: www.lesbianhealthinfo.org

Mautner Project: www.mautnerproject.org

National Sexuality Resource Center: www.nsrc.sfsu.edu

National Vulvodynia Association: www.nva.org

North American Menopause Society: www.menopause.org

Sexual Health Network: www.sexualhealth.com

Society for Sex Therapy and Research (SSTAR): www.sstarnet.org

Women's Sexual Health Foundation: www.twshf.org

Appendix

Barbach, L. *Pleasures: Women Write Erotica*. New York: Harper and Row, 1985.

Bloch, A., and Block, R., *Guide for Cancer Supporters*. Kansas City, MO: R. A. Bloch Cancer Foundation, Inc., 1995.

Heiman, J. R., and LoPiccolo, J. *Becoming Orgasmic: A Sexual and Personal Growth Program for Women*. New York: Prentice Hall, 1988.

Kroll, K., and Klein, E. L. *Enabling Romance: A Guide to Love, Sex, and Relationships for the Disabled (and the People Who Care About Them)*. New York: Harmony Books, 1992.

Ladas, A., Whipple, B., and Perry, J. *The G Spot: And Other Discoveries About Human Sexuality*. New York: Holt, 2004.

Laken, V., and Laken, K. *Making Love Again: Hope for Couples Facing Loss of Sexual Intimacy*. East Sandwich, MA: Ant Hill Press, 2002.

LaTour, K. *The Breast Cancer Companion*. New York: William Morrow and Co., 1994.

Pederson, L., and Trigg, J. M. *Breast Cancer: A Family Survival Guide*. Westport, CT: Greenwood Publishing, 1995.

Schover, L. *Sexuality and Fertility After Cancer*. New York: Wiley, 1997.

Valins, L. *When a Woman's Body Says No to Sex: Understanding and Overcoming Vaginismus*. New York: Penguin, 1992.

Zilbergeld, B. *The New Male Sexuality*, rev. ed. New York: Bantam, 1999.

Videotapes

Becoming Orgasmic: A Sexual and Personal Growth Program for Women. . . and the Men Who Love Them. Chapel Hill, NC: The Sinclair Institute, 1993.

A Man's Guide to Stronger Erections. Chapel Hill, NC: The Sinclair Institute, 1998.

Sex After 50. Fort Lauderdale, FL: Sex After 50, Inc., 1991.

Treating Vaginismus. Chapel Hill, NC: The Sinclair Institute, 1984.

Selected Websites and Telephone Numbers

Alexander Foundation for Women's Health: www.afwh.org

American Cancer Society: www.cancer.org, (800) ACS-2345

Cancer Care, Inc.: www.cancercare.org, (800) 813-4673

Centers for Disease Control and Prevention: www.cdc.gov/cancer,
    (888) 842-6355
Female Sexual Dysfunction: www.femalesexualdysfunctiononline.org
Impotence.org: www.impotence.org
International Society for Sexual and Impotence Research: www.issir.org
International Society for the Study of Women's Sexual Health: www.isswsh.org
Mautner Project for Lesbians with Cancer: www.mautnerproject.org,
    (202) 332-5536
National Council on Aging: www.ncoa.org
National Institute of Health: www.nih.gov
National Vulvodynia Association (USA): www.nva.org
Sexual Health.com: www.sexualhealth.com
Sexuality Information and Education Council of Canada: www.sieccan.org
Sexuality Information and Education Council of the U.S.: www.sieccus.org
Society for Sex Therapy and Research: www.sstarnet.org
Susan G. Komen Breast Cancer Foundation: www.komen.org,
    (800) IM-AWARE (1-800-462-9273)
Wellness Community: help@wellness-community.org or
    www.wellness-community.org, (888) 793-WELL

Ladies First: www.ladiesfirst.com. Wholesale manufacturer offers
    postmastectomy products including bras, camisoles, and active wear.
    More information: 800-497-8285; e-mail info@ladiesfirst.com

Lucy's Breast Forms: www.lucys.net. Purchase bras, breast forms, breast
    enhancers, attachable nipples, and accessories from different brands.
    More information: 866-264-9500 or 727-532-0330; e-mail lucys@lucys.net

Mastectomy.com: www.mastectomyshop.com. This postmastectomy boutique
    sells breast forms, bras, camisoles, swimsuits, lymph edema sleeves, wigs,
    turbans, nightgowns, and other apparel. You can also get fitted for your
    bra online.
    More information: 888-966-7068

New You Mastectomy Boutique: www.newyouboutique.com. Offers wide
    selection of mastectomy products. Lists products by brand.
    More information: 888-737-2511; e-mail newyou1@aol.com

Nicola Jane: www.nicolajane.com. This Europe-based store has a wide collection of modern-looking swimsuits, bras, and clothing. Sizes are listed according to United Kingdom standards, but the website includes a conversion chart. Prices converted upon purchase.
More information: info@nicolajane.com

www.nottiwear.com Covers lumpectomy and mastectomy scars as well as abdominal scars. Comes in variety of colors.
More information: feelsexy@nottiwear.com

Woman's Personal Health Source: www.womanspersonalhealth.com. Carries front-closure, compression, sports, leisure, and gel bras, as well as swimwear, back supports, and other mastectomy products.
More information: 877-463-1343; e-mail: wphinc@hotmail.com

Endocrinology
American Association of Endocrinologists: www.aace.com
Endocrine Society: www.endo-society.org

Therapist Links
American Association of Sex Educators, Counselors, and Therapists: www.assect.org/home/

Obstetrics/Gynecology
American College of Obstetricians and Gynecologists: www.acog.org
North American Menopausal Society (NAMS): www.menopause.org

Appendix

Glossary

A

Acupuncture: A traditional Chinese practice of treating a health condition or medical state by inserting needles into the skin at specific points to unblock the flow of energy.

Anorgasmia: Difficulty experiencing or the inability to experience orgasm; in women it is often referred to as female orgasmic disorder.

Antidepressant: The best medication to treat depression and panic attacks. Antidepressants are nonaddictive and may benefit the central nervous system in many ways.

Aphrodisiac: A substance believed to improve or enhance sexual function or pleasure. Some think it may stimulate feelings of love, intimacy, or desire.

Aromatase inhibitors: Drugs that suppress the body's natural production of estrogen by reducing production of the enzyme aromatase.

Aromatherapy: An integrative care practice that uses oils from plants to treat physical or psychological conditions. The oils can be inhaled, used in vaporizers, or used in massage.

Autoerotic: Providing sexual stimulation to oneself or being aroused sexually by oneself.

B

Bilateral salpingo-oophorectomy: The surgical term for the removal of both the right and left Fallopian tubes and ovaries.

Bimanual vaginal examination: Examination of the vagina, cervix, and uterus as well as the other internal pelvic organs with the use of gloved fingers that are inserted into the vagina while the other hand presses on the abdomen.

Bioidentical hormones: Hormonal preparations usually of animal or plant origin that have a similar structure to naturally occurring human hormones.

Biopsy: A surgical procedure that involves obtaining a tissue specimen from the body for laboratory testing to determine a more precise diagnosis.

C

Cancer: A disease characterized by uncontrolled cell growth that ultimately causes destruction of normal healthy tissue.

Cervix: From the Latin word meaning neck; it is the lower most part of the uterus that protrudes into the vagina.

Chlamydia infection: A sexually transmitted disease caused by the infection with the bacterium Chlamydia trachomatis.

Clitoris: The erectile organ in women; the external portion is located at the junction of the labia minora just in front of the vestibule.

Coitus: Latin word for the penetration of the vagina with a penis.

Colposcopy: A diagnostic procedure performed by gynecologists to examine the cervix more closely.

Contraception: The prevention of fertilization and pregnancy, usually with pills or other hormonal manipulation of the women's reproductive cycle. Sometimes intrauterine devices can be also used.

Cunnilingus: Sexual contact between the tongue or mouth of one person and the vulva/clitoral tissue of another.

D

Depression: A state of lowered mood usually associated with other disturbances such as sleep issues, loss of or uncontrollable appetite, and loss of life's pleasure. Serious cases may be associated with suicidal thoughts.

Dildo: A sexual toy that is often phallic in nature or shaped like a penis and that can be used to penetrate the vagina or anus. Both men and women often incorporate dildos into sexual play. Another term often used is vaginal/anal dilator.

Dopamine: A catecholamine that serves as a neurotransmitter and also as a hormone inhibiting the release of prolactin from the anterior portion of the pituitary gland. It is involved in

the neurochemistry of sexual function for both men and women.

Dyspareunia: Pain with sexual intercourse.

E

Erectile dysfunction: A persistent or recurrent inability to achieve or maintain an erection sufficient enough to accomplish a desired sexual behavior such as intercourse or coitus; earlier it was described as impotence.

Erection: The expansion and hardening or stiffening of the sexual organ; it may be the penis, clitoris, or nipples in response to sexual fantasy or stimulation.

Erotica: Sexually themed work such as books or sculpture deemed to have literary and artistic merit. Naked men, women, and other body parts are often featured as predominant themes.

Estrogen: A steroid hormone produced mainly in the ovaries; the primary female sexual hormone.

F

Fellatio: Latin word for the sexual act between the mouth of one person and the penis of another.

Female androgen insufficiency syndrome: A constellation of symptoms attributed to low testosterone levels in women. Some of the symptoms include fatigue, decreased well-being, lack of energy or motivation, and decreased or absent sexual interest or desire.

Female circumcision: Any form of ritualized genital cutting or excision or destruction of parts of the female genitalia.

Female ejaculation: Expulsion from the urethra in women of about 3 to 5 milliliters of fluid different in chemical composition from urine.

Fibroid: A benign tumor arising from smooth muscle cells of the uterus.

Food and Drug Administration (FDA): Federal agency that protects public health by regulating the safety and efficacy of food, medical products, biotechnology, and cosmetics. No drug or device can be sold on the market unless it has undergone vigorous scientific testing and passed the strict regulations of the FDA.

Foreplay: Sexual behavior engaged in during the early part of the sexual encounter, with the aim at intensifying sexual arousal or pleasure.

G

Glans: The terminal knob of the penis or clitoris.

Gräfenberg spot (G-spot): An area of increased erotic sensitivity on or deep in the front of the vagina. It is located on the anterior surface of the vaginal vault. Stimulation in some women provides intense sexual pleasure.

H

Hormone therapy: The use of medications to modify or replace hormones that are decreased or absent in the menopause period.

Hypertension: High blood pressure. An abnormality in arterial blood pressure that typically results from a thickening of the blood vessel wall. It is a risk factor for many illnesses including heart attacks, heart failure, and stroke or end-stage kidney disease.

Hyperthyroidism: Increased thyroid hormone production that can cause symptoms such as anxiety, weight loss, and at times can mimic panic attacks.

Hysterectomy: Surgical removal of the uterus.

K

Kegel exercises: Exercises designed to increase muscle strength and elasticity in the pelvis. They may be recommended in the treatment of urinary incontinence.

L

Letrozole: An anti-estrogen-type of medication in the class of aromatase inhibitors. It inhibits the conversion of testosterone to estrogens.

Libido: Sexual interest or desire.

Lubrication: The natural appearance of slippery secretions in the vagina during sexual arousal or the use of artificial lubricants to facilitate sexual activity or intercourse.

M

Mammogram: A special X-ray of the breast tissue that can be used as a screening tool for breast cancer.

Mastectomy: The removal of the breast.

Masturbation: The act of self-pleasuring; also known as self-stimulation.

Glossary

Meditation: A complementary medicine practice of concentrated attention toward a single point of reference.

Menopause: The lack of menstrual cycles for one year; the permanent end of a woman's menstrual cycle.

Menstruation: Vaginal bleeding resulting from endometrial shedding following ovulation when the egg is not fertilized.

Monogamy: Sexually exclusive couple who do not have sexual relations with other people outside their relationship.

Mucosa: A surface layer of cells or epithelium that is lubricated by the secretions of mucosal glands.

O

Orgasm: The intense pleasurable sensation at the peak of sexual activity or sexual climax usually associated with spasmodic contraction of the pelvic floor muscles. It is often associated with ejaculation, especially in men.

Osteoporosis A condition characterized by decrease in bone mass and density of the bones resulting in "thinning" of the bones causing them to become more fragile.

Outercourse: Sexual activities other than intercourse; fondling, touching, kissing, oral and genital play are often considered outercourse. It can be promoted as a means of sexual activity that prevents unwanted pregnancy and that can minimize sexually transmitted diseases.

Ovulation: The process of egg release from the ovary.

P

Penis: The erectile, sexually, erotically sensitive organ in males. The penis serves a sexual function and also mediates the voiding of urine.

Perimenopause: The time in which women are having irregular periods before the periods completely stop. It can be several years in duration and is characterized by menopausal and nonmenopausal symptomatology.

Pheromone: A volatile compound released by one organism that triggers a specific behavior in another member of the same species.

Progesterone: A hormone that is secreted by the ovary and placenta (during pregnancy); it is necessary for pregnancy and has been implicated in female sexual function.

Progestin: A synthetic form of progesterone often used in birth control pills and hormone therapy.

Pubic hair: Hair that appears on portions of the external genitalia in both sexes at puberty.

S

Serotonin reuptake inhibitor: A type of depressant medication that does not allow serotonin to be taken up again by the neuroreceptors, thereby causing more serotonin to be present in the neuron. These may be used for depression and panic attacks.

Sexual intercourse (intercourse): Sexual contact usually involving coitus or penile vaginal penetration.

Sexuality: The feelings, behaviors, and identities associated with sex.

Sildenafil: A phosphodiesterase inhibitor that is used in the treatment of male erectile dysfunction. New data suggest this class of medication can sometimes be used for the treatment of serotonin reuptake inhibitor–induced female sexual problems.

T

Tamoxifen: A selective estrogen receptor modulator that is used in the treatment of breast cancer.

Tantra: An ancient Indian spiritual tradition and belief system with the premise that sexuality is tied into personal energy and is capable of changing us if we submit to our primal sexual desires while maintaining control and heightening spiritual awareness. Tantra can intensify lovemaking and intensify the sexual dynamic or consciousness between couples.

Testosterone: A sexual hormone that is produced in the ovaries and adrenal glands that is important in normal sexual functioning. It has been implicated in normal female libido or desire.

Topical anesthetics: Medication applied to the surface of the body, for example, the skin or mucous membrane, to numb the area.

U

Uterus: The female reproductive organ in which a pregnancy occurs.

V

Vagina: The part of the female genital tract that connects the uterus to the external vulva. It is 8 to 10 cm in length.

Vaginal atrophy: When the vaginal tissues decrease in size, become pale or dry and without lubrication; this is a result of decreased hormonal levels in the woman's body. The tissues can become sensitive and often vaginal atrophy is associated with painful intercourse. Commonly seen in chemical or natural menopause.

Vaginal dilators: Medical applications that can be placed within the vagina to help restore the vaginal tissues so that they are more adaptable.

Vaginismus: An involuntary tightening of the vaginal muscles when the vagina is penetrated. The action can cause significant distress and pain.

Vaginitis: Inflammation of the vagina.

Vulva: The external female genitals also commonly known as the vulvar lips.

Vulvodynia: Chronic painful irritation of the introitus or nearby tissues.

Y

Yoga: The spiritual practice aiming to unite the consciousness with universal consciousness to achieve harmony.

Yohimbine: An alkaloid medicine derived from the South American plant Corynanthe yohimbe, which has alleged aphrodisiac properties.

Index

Index

Index

Index